FAILURE TO FIND FAILURE TO THRIVE:

the case for improving screening, prevention and treatment in primary care

JANE BATCHELOR & ANDREW KERSLAKE

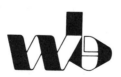

Whiting & Birch Ltd
London

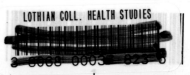

FAILURE TO FIND FAILURE TO THRIVE

the case for improving screening, prevention and treatment in primary care

© Jane Batchelor and Andrew Kerslake

All rights reserved. No reproduction, copy or transmission of this
publication may be made without written permission from the publishers

London 1990

Published by Whiting & Birch Ltd, PO Box 872, London SE23 3HL.

British Library Cataloguing in Publication Data
A CIP catalogue record in available from the British Library

ISBN 1 871177 05 7

Cover illustration by Katy Davies, age 6

Contents

ACKNOWLEDGEMENT

We wish to thank The Children's Society who commissioned the research, and the many health and social services personnel who made themselves available to us. We are especially grateful to the health visitors who willingly laid their work open to our scrutiny.

Jane Batchelor
Andrew Kerslake
November 1989

Introduction

In the early part of the twentieth century, the agenda for child health care in the Western World focused on overcoming poverty and malnutrition, and reducing the number of infant and child deaths through contagious diseases. In 1900 the infant mortality rate in England was 142 per thousand live births, but by 1946 it had been reduced to 42.7, and it is now down to about 9 per thousand live births (Central Statistical Office 1989). However, the death of Dennis O'Neill in the mid 1940s (O'Neill 1945) shifted the focus of child care on to child abuse. This has been the agenda throughout the latter part of the twentieth century.

Practice and research attention in the fields of child welfare have increasingly concentrated on physical and, of late, sexual abuse in comparison to failure to thrive (Drotar 1985). This is in contrast to the Third World where there is a body of research on the effects of malnutrition, and on screening procedures for children at risk (Briend & Bari 1989). This apparent lack of interest in the Western World may be due to a belief that nourishment problems in childhood, usually associated with poverty, no longer occur in significant numbers. Skuse (1988) suggests that young children who are provided with insufficient quantities of foods are "...likely to become stunted, yet their bodily proportions will remain approximately normal". This also applies to children who are provided with appropriate quantities of food but for some reason do not consume it. As a result, undernourished children may not be identified as part of the failure to thrive population, being misdiagnosed as children who are constitutionally small.

This publication is based on the findings from two studies of children under five who were failing to thrive. The research was commissioned by The Children's Society who wished to develop a project for such children. This work was undertaken within one specific geographical area where the project would be located. The research was designed to identify children who had failed to thrive over a given time period, to examine any interventions used and the outcome of those interventions. The aim was to develop indicators of failure to thrive so that particular children could be targeted for intervention, and to devise a model for a project providing effective treatment.

We knew from other research conducted in the same geographical area that failure to thrive rarely featured in social services records. From early discussions with health professionals it emerged that paediatric records were not stored in a manner that enabled children failing to thrive to be readily identified. As a consequence we had to find alternative child health data in order to locate these children.

We chose health visitors as the most appropriate source of information for identifying children for our studies. The National Health Service Act (1946) conferred on local health authorities the duty to provide health visitors "...for the purpose of giving advice as to the care of young children". Health visitors still make a priority of work with young children. In fulfilling their tasks of promoting health and preventing ill-health, developmental surveillance constitutes a large component of their practice. There is no nationally agreed screening system, nor a national directive that places an obligation on health visitors to weigh children. It is, however, the customary means by which health visitors monitor children's development. This monitoring is done in two ways. Firstly, health visitors have contact with children and mothers at child health clinics or at home. The frequency of this contact varies, depending on the manner in which health visitors choose to prioritise their work, and the level of use of child health clinics that parents choose to make. Secondly, health visitors and clinical medical officers undertake formal screening of pre-school children's development at certain ages, as determined by their health authority. In this manner they follow children's development from birth through to starting school.

The study area comprised one district of a local authority social services department in the south of England. Its boundaries are co-terminus with a district health authority. There are a number of small market towns and many villages in this predominately rural county; no major conurbations fell within the district studied. The area had an estimated population of 12,600 children under five in 1987, according to the local authority structure plan. This population was served by 51 health visitors, some employed on a part-time basis.

The criteria for inclusion in each study were that the child had been on or below the 3rd centile for weight in 1987 and was aged under five at that time. The first sample was drawn from 21 health visitors' caseloads, on the basis of the health visitors' recall of children fitting the study criteria. The second sample was obtained by examination of child health records from the remaining 30 health visitors' caseloads. Existing studies of failure to thrive show a prevalence rate of between 1% and 9% of the child population. Therefore between 120 and 1,100 children in the study area could have been expected to fit our research criteria.

The research was conducted at a time when the social services department and the health authority were both addressing issues relating to services for under fives. The district health authority had recently reviewed screening procedures. The social services department had commissioned research which looked at the process by which children were admitted to care. It was also at the point of revising its criteria for priority day care for children. Finally, a rapid growth in the number of under fives in the area was anticipated, due to planned population growth.

Section 1

The failure to thrive literature

1. DEFINITIONS AND PREVALENCE OF FAILURE TO THRIVE

One factor that is common to all children described as failing to thrive is that they are, for whatever reason, undernourished and not receiving adequate nutrition for normal growth (Skuse 1988). Normal growth is usually defined in relative terms. Centile charts allow a child's growth to be viewed in relation to the growth of a 'normal' population. Tanner and Whitehouse (1959) used data from a number of large-scale studies of children's growth to develop growth centile charts. These are now widely used in child health clinics in Britain.

Charts are available to plot children's weight, height and head circumference over time. Taking the weight centile chart as an example (Figure 1), the axes of the chart are weight (in kilos) and age (in months or years). Onto the chart are printed several centile lines; usually the 3rd, 10th, 50th, 90th and 97th. Each line is drawn on the basis of data on weight-for-age from these large-scale studies. The 50th centile is the line connecting points at which, for that age, 50% of children would be below that weight and 50% above. The 3rd centile is the line connecting points at which only 3% of children would be below that weight and 97% above.

A child's weight at different ages can be plotted onto a centile chart, and the points joined to give a line showing that child's weight gain, or loss, over time. This line can then be compared to those printed on the centile chart. The charts are valuable as a tool for identifying children who are deviating from their growth pattern, crossing centile lines. The most thorough assessment can be made when charts for weight, height and head circumference have been completed. As the report, "A Child in Trust" (Beckford 1985) describes:

> Once the child has reached the age of 4 months and has established
> a pattern of growth, he [sic] is likely to remain on the centile. If the

Figure 1. Weight Centile Chart

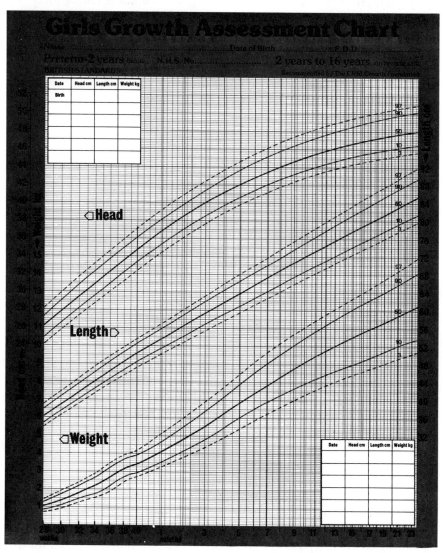

The growth chart was compiled by Dr D. Gairdner and Julie Pearson, and first described in *Archives of Disease in Childhood*, Vol 46. p783. As a clinical chart, its publication reference is GPG3 and is reproduced in chart reference 22A as part of a complete Growth Assessment record. Castlemead Publications have the copyright license and it is reproduced here with permission.

chart then shows that the child's weight or height is falling away from the centile formerly followed, alarm bells should start ringing (p72).

Thus the extent to which a child is following an established pattern of growth can be determined from centile charts. Some children will be born small and remain small, establishing a growth pattern that follows a low centile line. It is to be expected that approximately 3% of children will be below the 3rd centile, by virtue of the way the charts are constructed. However, the 3rd centile is commonly used as a means of identifying children at risk since, if a child has established an earlier growth pattern closer to the norm (eg, above the 10th centile) then a drop to the 3rd centile represents a potentially serious deviation. Loss of weight or reduction in rate of weight gain can be an early indicator of a range of adverse conditions, both medical and social.

Knowing that a child is below the 3rd centile for weight does not necessarily mean the child is of absolute low weight; nor does it necessarily mean that the child is not thriving. What it does tell us is that, relative to the population of children whose weights were used for constructing the centile charts, such children are of low weight. If charts were constructed on the basis of a sample of children in a country with considerable poverty, then in terms of their absolute weights we might have good reason to be concerned about all children below the 50th centile.

Beyond the common factor of low weight for age, the diagnosis of failure to thrive has been applied to children exhibiting a range of conditions (Oates 1984; Lachenmeyer & Davidovicz 1987). The diagnosis of organic failure to thrive is applied to children for whom an organic base to their low weight is found. When no such condition is found then non-organic or environmental failure to thrive is diagnosed. This latter diagnosis may rest on the child having gained weight whilst in hospital for investigation of low weight. Failure to thrive has also been defined in terms of the lack of overall growth, eg, below the 3rd centile for height in addition to weight. It may or may not include developmental delay. Articles and research studies describing children who are failing to thrive often use different definitions and, in some, these are not made explicit. These differences in definition may account for the wide variations in prevalence rates, as we describe below.

Various studies have attempted to estimate the extent of failure to thrive in the Western World. These have drawn their samples from different populations of children; hospital in-patients, out-patients, users of primary health care and inner-city children; obviously this makes comparison difficult. In addition, findings from studies undertaken in the USA need to be interpreted with caution when applied to Britain. Different health care systems operate in the two countries, so identification rates may be based on very different populations.

Lachenmeyer and Davidovicz (1987), in their review article, quote two studies on prevalence rates based on in-patient populations. The first reported that between 3% and 5% of all infants under 1 year of age admitted to paediatric teaching hospitals are diagnosed as cases of failure to thrive, whilst the second found that 1% of all cases admitted to paediatric hospitals are identified as failing to thrive, with 80% of cases being infants younger than 18 months. Skuse (1985) cites studies that suggest between 1% and 5% of paediatric admissions are of children failing to thrive, and that less than one quarter of these children have an organic disease. In an out-patient setting Smithells (1982) reviewed the diagnostic indices of his outpatient paediatric appointments and found that 2% were infants whose growth was delayed, including failure to thrive. A further 6% had problems of feeding, or vomiting and diarrhoea.

Turning to the primary care setting, Mitchell et al (1980) followed a cohort of 312 children in three rural primary care settings in North Carolina, USA. They identified 30 children with non-organic failure to thrive, giving an incidence rate in the primary care setting of 9.6%. Finally, Skuse (1988) quotes a figure of up to 5% of infants born in inner-city communities in Britain failing to thrive. Recent unpublished research by the same author suggests the proportion of such infants with an organic disease or disorder is about 6%.

2. THE CONSEQUENCES OF FAILING TO THRIVE

Within the Third World, health professionals are often dealing with children for whom the direct consequence of their failure to thrive may be death. In such a setting we assume their focus will be on differentiating between those children who will live (albeit with retarded growth), those who would die without immediate intervention, and those who are beyond help. Such basic differentiation is vital in a setting where resources are severely limited, and where many children suffer from such extreme malnutrition that death is a frequent consequence.

In the developed world, health professionals are rarely faced with such situations. Only occasionally do children die as a direct result of failure to thrive. Such children are not part of a starving population for whom insufficient food is available, as found in the Third World. These children have been starved by a parent; extreme neglect has resulted in the child not being fed, despite food being available. In addition, some abused children who die as a result of their injuries are found to have been failing to thrive (Beckford 1985; Carlile 1987). Therefore, whilst death from failure to thrive can occur in the Western World, it appears that this is not the reason that screening for low weight is undertaken. The importance of identifying failure to thrive rests on other risks. Firstly, it may result in permanent damage, secondly, it may be associated with developmental delay and, finally, failure to thrive may act as an indicator of other problems, including abuse and neglect.

Immediate physical effects

There is evidence to suggest a child's growth, including development of the brain, may be permanently impaired as a consequence of failure to thrive. Factors such as the child's age and the length of the failure to thrive episode are important variables that may ameliorate or exacerbate these effects, although the evidence regarding the extent of catch-up growth that may be achieved is not conclusive.

There are important physiological factors that make young children especially vulnerable if they receive inadequate nutrition. As Taylor and Taylor (1976) state:

> The period between the start of weaning and the fifth birthday is nutritionally the most vulnerable segment of the human life cycle. Rapid growth, loss of passive immunity and as yet undeveloped acquired immunity against infection produce dietary needs more specific and inflexible than at later periods (p82).

Children's limited fat stores mean that their reserves are depleted very quickly. In periods of undernutrition their bodies then adapt by curtailment of the growth process. This may result in a reduction of cell number or cell size, both being means by which the body preserves essential cell function (Winick 1980).

Children who have been admitted to hospital with non-organic failure to thrive have consistently shown "..a substantially increased risk of continued growth retardation" (Skuse 1985). Likewise Haynes et al (1983), in the introduction to a study of 16 hospitalised infants diagnosed as failing to thrive, summarise findings from earlier studies that demonstrate failure to thrive can result in permanent damage to physical growth and all aspects of development, or even death if untreated. Failure to thrive is therefore important as children who do not receive adequate nutrition when young may always have limited growth. It may also have other permanent effects. Undernourished children are at greater risk of contracting illnesses (Lobstein 1988). Differences in infant feeding may also determine subsequent differences in adult mortality (Barker & Osmond 1987).

Illingworth (1983) refers to evidence of malnutrition inflicting damage to the brain if not corrected in the early weeks of infancy. He also cites work by Cravioto who found that recovery from malnutrition was only accompanied by mental improvement if the children's episode of severe malnourishment commenced after the age of 6 months. Illingworth (1983) concludes by saying:

Studies all over the world have shown that severe growth retardation in the first year retards later mental development, and the longer the duration of the growth retardation, the greater is the effect on mental development (p39).

Pacey and Payne (1985) point to the relationships between body size and various functions such as immunity to disease and mental functioning. Whilst it is known that these functions are interrelated, the links between them are not yet well understood. Pacey and Payne quote studies which have established an association between severe malnutrition and poor mental development, but not a direct causal link. For example, several studies have shown that malnutrition stunts brain size, whilst others show that children who suffer severe protein-energy malnutrition score poorly on IQ tests. However, there may be a range of factors which result in poor performance on such tests. Pacey and Payne (1985) conclude, "...if there were a causal relationship between malnutrition and reduced mental development, it would be a very complex one".

The extent to which children may achieve catch-up growth is still a matter of debate. Factors such as the child's age and the length of the failure to thrive episode are important variables. MacCarthy (1974) concludes that short periods of severe malnutrition "...do not appear to preclude the attainment of normal height, weight and build in later childhood". This begs the question, how short is a 'short period' of severe malnutrition? Prader (1978) writes that "...a growth deficit acquired in late gestation or during infancy is usually followed by a complete or near complete catch-up growth, provided the growth deficiency is not too severe or too long", yet he does not specify what 'too severe' and 'too long' mean. Finally, Oates (1984) reviews the findings of six follow-up studies of failure to thrive children from which he concludes "...catch-up growth following non-organic failure to thrive seems to occur in the majority of children". However, the studies he quotes show a wide variation both in time elapsed prior to follow-up (from 1 to 11 years) and in the percentage of study children who were above the 3rd centile for weight on follow-up (from 86% down to 32%). In contrast, regarding the effects of chronic undernutrition and undernourishment, Skuse (1988) writes:

> There is some evidence that if a growth trajectory is established within the first year of life such that both weight and length are in proportion, but at the lower limit of or below the normal range, the body's capacity for subsequent catch-up growth is curtailed (p6).

In conclusion, children can suffer permanent damage as a result of failure to thrive. Despite the lack of an established causal link, studies suggest that the earlier the malnutrition, the worse the retardation of physical and intellectual development. They also indicate that recovery may be possible for some children in the long-term, through catch-up growth. However, whether or not the association subsequently disappears is likely to depend on the child's age and the extent of the failure to thrive episode.

Secondary impairments associated with failure to thrive

Studies of environmentally-based (non-organic) failure to thrive illustrate long term psychological effects, such as more behaviour problems among failure to thrive children than comparison groups, as cited by Drotar (1985), and high rates of behavioural disturbance among school aged children (Hufton & Oates 1977). However, the lack of certainty about developmental delay as a cause or a consequence of failure to thrive is highlighted in a cohort study of 312 children in primary care centres in the USA (Mitchell et al

1980). The researchers were interested in whether current behavioural and developmental deficits of the children were attributable to failure to thrive, rather than to social conditions coinciding with failure to thrive. From their follow-up examination of 19 cases and 19 controls they concluded that the developmental deficits were not a consequence of failure to thrive, but rather that social stresses in the family were more likely to be the cause of the developmental deficits which were seen both in children with failure to thrive and in those with normal growth. Thus it may be that both failure to thrive and developmental delay are caused by the same environmental or family factors rather than failure to thrive causing developmental delay or vice versa. Mitchell et al (1980) write:

> The alarm with which failure to thrive is often viewed is probably not justified on the basis of potential sequelae of the failure to thrive, except as an indication of situational problems which may be damaging to the child regardless of his growth status (p976).

Failure to thrive as an indicator of other problems

Failure to thrive may be an indicator of other medical, social or 'situational problems' (Mitchell et al 1980). Children may be in receipt of a poor diet because they live in poverty, or because their parents do not know about the dietary needs of growing children. These issues can be addressed, at least in part, by primary health care teams through education and welfare rights advice. Weight loss or poor weight gain may be an indicator that a child is suffering from an undiagnosed, possibly life-threatening, organic condition. For example, children suffering from cystic fibrosis have major problems with digestion, resulting in poor growth. Failure to thrive is important to health professionals since early identification can result in detection of a previously undiagnosed organic condition that requires treatment.

Failure to thrive is also perceived as an indicator of potential child abuse. It has been visible in children who have died through abuse, and Laking (1988) suggests a significant proportion of abused children have failed to thrive prior to being subjected to abuse. However, Skuse (1988) argues that failure to thrive "...is not usually associated with child abuse or neglect". Some failure to thrive children are neglected or abused; some neglected or abused children fail to thrive. The failure to thrive, when it occurs, may be a cause or a consequence of the abuse or neglect. The two populations overlap, but the extent of, and reasons for, the overlap are still a matter of debate.

Failure to thrive may indicate that feeding problems exist. Such problems were examined in studies by Iwaniec et al (1985, 1985b, 1988). Whether feeding problems are a cause or a consequence of a particular child's failure to thrive, they may escalate if the child is subsequently diagnosed as not having an organic base for the failure to thrive. This risk may be highest if the child has readily accepted food and gained weight whilst in hospital. Parents may feel irritated and dissatisfied with such a child, and the child in turn can become increasingly attention-seeking and demanding. Others have referred to the spiral that can develop between an angry, hungry child and a tense, tired parent (Laking 1988).

In conclusion, death is now rarely a consequence of failure to thrive in the developed world. However, failure to thrive can result in impaired growth and development, and as the potential for catch-up growth has its limits, the effects can be far-reaching. Finally, failure to thrive can be useful as a potential indicator of other problems a child and its family are experiencing. The relationship is likely to be interactive; failure to thrive may usefully be viewed as part of a spiral of difficulties rather than as a cause or a consequence of other problems.

3. WHO FAILS TO THRIVE

Potential indicators of children failing to thrive fall into four categories: poverty and environment, parental behaviour, the child's behaviour and parent-child interaction.

It is clear that poverty alone, in Western societies, is not an indicator of a child failing to thrive (Gagan et al 1984, Forfar & Arneil 1984). Children suffering from failure to thrive are found in families from all socio- economic groups, and not all poor children fail to thrive. However, level of disposable income will have a bearing on diet. Parents who are living on a very low income have a limited choice of diet open to them (Lobstein 1988). Nutrition surveys undertaken in the USA in the 1970s all link poverty to diets of inadequate quality and quantity (Frank et al 1985). Only a small amount (12.7g/day) of protein is necessary for growth for children aged 1 to 3 years (MacCarthy 1974). However, a child's diet may be deficient in areas other than protein; for example, calorie intake may be too low for the child's needs. In such cases the body will use protein to supply the necessary calories. Thus what would have been a protein intake sufficient for growth can be insufficient, if used for calories.

The research on parental behaviour tends to focus on two themes; general behaviour and neglect. Several studies conclude that there is no link between psychopathology of parents (in this case mothers) and failure to thrive (Pollitt et al 1975, Kotelchuck 1980, Iwaniec et al 1985). However, it has been suggested that mothers of children who are failing to thrive are socially disadvantaged in various ways, tending to score relatively highly on measures of anxiety and depression and low on measures of self-esteem (Iwaniec et al 1985). Also mothers of failure to thrive children have been described as having "inoperant" maternal behaviour (Pollitt et al 1975), on the basis that it differed substantially from that of mothers of thriving children.

The finding of maternal isolation is a common one in studies of mothers of failure to thrive children. For example, Kotelchuck (1980) noted that mothers of such children were isolated from marital, familial, and neighbourhood support. Gagan et al (1984) explored the characteristics of social support among families of 55 children under 30 months who had been diagnosed as failing to thrive (44 non-organic and 11 organic). Their research findings supported the hypothesis that mothers of failure to thrive children do not have good social support networks.

Two factors associated with failure to thrive children are prematurity and low birth weight (Farnaroff & Klaus 1972, Lachenmeyer & Davidovicz 1987). Between 10% and 40% of children in the USA hospitalised for failure to thrive were low birth weight, compared to 7% of all newborns (Frank et al 1985). There is a possible link with poverty here, as low income mothers are at increased risk of bearing low birth weight babies. Kotelchuck (1980) cites studies showing that "...the infant's physical and social characteristics often directly contribute to his own malnutrition". Malnourished and premature infants are less vigorous in their sucking, putting them at risk of becoming part of a "cycle of interactive failure" (Kotelchuck 1980). If a baby is unresponsive and sickly then it may be slower to evoke caretaking behaviour from parents. Thus child-related factors and not maternal factors may be the most important risk indicators of growth retardation.

Some studies have looked at links between neglect and failure to thrive (Kotelchuck 1980; Bithoney & Newberger 1987). Both conclude that there is little evidence to suggest that failure to thrive is caused by neglectful parents. However, one study begins to explore ideas which lead to a third set of indicators, that of the child's birth or behaviour. Bithoney and Newberger (1987) conclude that their sample was characterised by "a striking prevalence of temperamental and behavioural aberration in children with failure to thrive". The children were described as more sickly and behaviourally difficult than matched controls, with a significantly higher reactivity and distractibility to extraneous stimuli. They suggest that the children's below-age locomotive skills, more highly variable 'tempo of play' and increased 'fussiness' might also add to the frustration and disappointed expectations often inherent in caring for a small, sick, temperamentally-delayed infant. However, they also make the point that temperamental aberrations may be due to malnutrition, as has been found in studies undertaken in the Third World.

It has been suggested that personality traits of infants failing to thrive fall into two extreme categories (Gagan et al 1984). They are either irritable, hyperactive and difficult to comfort, or lethargic, slow-moving and undemanding. Skuse (1985) refers to a study by Leonard in the 1960s in which it was found that mothers with demanding growth-retarded babies were often tense and anxious whereas slow apathetic infants tended to be ignored. In looking at the temperamental patterns of children in their study, Iwaniec et al (1985) found the index group displayed more of the attributes categorised as 'difficult' or 'slow to warm up' than the contrast children. They write:

> The children's patterns of unmalleable behaviour, resistance to new routines.....and their general volatility of mood and behaviour, appeared to make them difficult to rear from early in life. Feeding routines, and other training tasks, were made into fraught enterprises for many parents (p258).

However, the range of behaviours exhibited by children failing to thrive cannot occur in isolation from either the environment or parents/caregivers. Therefore, the final potential territory for indicators is parent-child interaction. A day-to-day activity that necessitates such interaction, and is central to weight gain and growth, is feeding.

Some studies have directly addressed the feeding behaviour of failure to thrive children. For example, although Kotelchuck's own study (1980) failed to discover particular feeding difficulties in failure to thrive infants he cites two earlier studies that reported that parents of failure to thrive children had more feeding problems with their children than did matched controls. Iwaniec et al (1985) state that all parents in the index group in their study of failure to thrive children reported specific feeding difficulties in their children, and that feeding time appeared to be a period of heightened stress for mothers. They go on to make an interesting observation on the way 'treatment' can exacerbate the problem. In their research all children were admitted to hospital at the outset of the study and any organic base for their failure to thrive excluded. This apparently resulted in parents expecting the feeding problems to disappear since they thought there was no reason for the child to reject food, and so the battles with their children around feeding escalated.

4. CONCLUSIONS FROM THE LITERATURE

This review of the research literature tells us several things of importance concerning children who are failing to thrive. Firstly, whilst definitions of failure to thrive vary, the most common indicator used is that of children being below the 3rd centile for weight. Whilst this is a relative measure there is sufficient evidence of both immediate and long term ill-effects for it to still have an absolute value. Secondly, although failure to thrive appears to have dropped from attention, the numbers of children for whom this may be a serious condition are not insignificant. Thirdly, whilst several sources speak of the harm and damage caused to children, we are unable to discover material that precisely links age of incidence and extent of the failure to thrive episode with eventual consequences and outcome. Fourthly, explanations of failure to thrive in terms of links with poverty, neglect, developmental delay or child abuse, whilst present in various cases, are not capable either individually or collectively of acting as indicators. However, certain factors related to feeding, nutrition and parent-child interaction look to be more fruitful avenues to explore.

Section 2

The first failure to thrive study

1. BACKGROUND TO THE FIRST STUDY

We decided to use weight on or below the 3rd centile as the primary criterion for selection of our study sample for two reasons. Firstly, from our reading of the literature we had found this to be the one factor common to all definitions of failure to thrive. Secondly, we knew that weighing children was one way that health visitors maintained surveillance of children's growth and development and that children's weights were recorded by health visitors.

Initially we planned to study only those children for whom no organic basis for their weight loss or poor weight gain had been found; ie, those who had been diagnosed as suffering from non-organic failure to thrive. Children suffering from organic failure to thrive were dealt with in the literature as requiring medical identification and treatment, not the services of a failure to thrive project. However, as our reading progressed it became clear that separating organic from non-organic was a false distinction, since the conditions are not mutually exclusive. A child can suffer from an organic condition, resulting in a diagnosis of organic failure to thrive, whilst at the same time be failing to thrive for non-organic reasons. For example, a child with Down's Syndrome might have poor growth as a result of a heart condition. At the same time, if parents experience difficulties in coming to terms with their child's handicap, day-to-day interaction with the child may be full of tension. In such an environment mealtimes can quickly become a battle ground, resulting in the child not eating and so failing to thrive for non-organic reasons. We also decided not to exclude premature or low birth weight babies from the study, since the existing research pointed to the part a child could play in its own failure to thrive. For example, a premature baby fed by tube in a special care baby unit may not develop the usual ability to suck. This could lead to later feeding difficulties and slow weight gain which are only in part directly attributable to the baby's low birth weight.

Finally, we recognised from the literature that traditional medical diagnosis divided children who were failing to thrive into organic or non-organic. If we were to develop indicators enabling us to target our population more closely we would need to establish some common patterns, within these diagnoses, to the failure to thrive episodes. We hypothesised that patterns of failure to thrive might follow one of three courses.

Constants

This group would drop below the 3rd centile and then stay beneath it. Some would make small weight gains, sufficient for them not to dive far below the centile, but not sufficient to climb above it. They were likely to be suffering from chronic, low-level undernutrition that may result in all-round stunted growth, so that they might be below the third centile for height as well as weight. As such they could easily be misdiagnosed as small rather than failing to thrive. Such children would cause less anxiety to health professionals than the other two groups, even though the effects of such failure to thrive might be far reaching.

Divers

This group would suddenly and progressively lose weight (or fail to gain) and dive down the centile chart, rapidly crossing the centile lines. Such children were likely to have a totally organic base to their failure to thrive. If the condition was one that would respond to treatment then once such treatment was started their weight gain would soon be back on course.

Dippers

This group would dip down and up, crossing and recrossing the 3rd centile. Some dips might be the direct result of several short-term organic conditions, such as bronchitis or vomiting and diarrhoea. Others might be associated with family stress around such issues as a parent experiencing feeding problems with the child, illness of other family members or breakdown of family relationships. Weight gain would follow treatment or intervention (eg, intensive health visitor input, or hospital admission). However, the gain would stop when intervention ceased and the child would again dip below the 3rd centile. In other words, regular intervention ensured these children climbed above the 3rd centile from time to time, only to drop back below it once the intervention ceased. Such children, if detected, would be likely to cause most anxiety to health professionals, since treatment did not 'cure' the failure to thrive, and constant surveillance would be necessary.

2. THE RESEARCH DESIGN AND PROCESS

We chose health visitors as our source of data on children failing to thrive, since they have extensive knowledge of the pre-school population. A total of 51 health visitors worked in the area. We knew the estimated under-fives population for the area was over 12,000. Given the time available for the research it was not possible for us to search all records to identify children below the 3rd centile. Therefore we relied on health visitor recall. Thus we confined ourselves to the 21 health visitors who had been in post for least 18 months and were available for interview at the time of the research.

Before conducting individual interviews, we held two group discussions with health visitors and their managers (Community Nurse Specialists). These discussions helped to clarify which children caused greatest concern for health visitors and why. They also helped us in constructing the two questionnaires we used in the individual health visitor interviews. The first questionnaire (see Appendix I) was designed to obtain a profile of each health visitor's caseload and of her working environment, including resources for children failing to thrive. The second (see Appendix II) was completed for each child under five whom health visitors recalled as on or below the 3rd centile for weight in 1987. This was completed through discussion and examination of each child's clinic notes. In addition to basic demographic data, information was recorded on the course of events since concern was first expressed about the child's weight, including treatment and outcome. The research interviews were conducted at least one year after the children had been below the 3rd centile, allowing sufficient time to have elapsed for identification and treatment of the failure to thrive to have occurred.

We were aware of drawbacks to this research design. We were not looking at caseloads where there had been a recent change of health visitor. We had to rely on each health visitor's recall, from her caseload of under-fives (often 200-300), of those children that had fallen onto the 3rd centile (often only 2 or 3). Since health visitors have far more frequent contact with babies than they do with toddlers, we hypothesised they would recall the youngest failure to thrive children most readily. Finally, although health visitors see the majority of children under five, a few are not brought to clinics by their parents and so could slip through the health visitor 'net'.

However, we had reason to believe that limitations of recall might not be extensive. The research took place during a time when weight charts had a high profile in the health authority and standardisation of developmental screening of children meant there was an emphasis on completion of charts for children's weight, height and head circumference. Many health visitors had undertaken recent additional training in this area.

Time did not allow us to extract additional data on the failure to thrive children from hospital or social services records. However, we did discuss with social services staff projected figures for under-fives in the area, existing provision for this age group and proposals for new developments. We also interviewed a range of health service staff about provision of services.

3. FINDINGS FROM THE FIRST STUDY

Our findings can be divided into two areas. Firstly, there is material from health visitor group discussions and from the individual interviews, about their work environment and general issues relating to failure to thrive children. The themes and topics covered in the group discussions and interviews ranged from general factors that influence health visitor practice in all areas of work to issues specific to failure to thrive children and their needs. They fell into seven areas. Secondly, we have quantitative data on the children identified as meeting the research criteria.

Training and experience of health visitors interviewed

Amongst the 21 health visitors interviewed, there was a wide range of experience. Half had been qualified for more than ten years, but 6 of the 21 had been qualified for under four years. Of those interviewed, 85% had undertaken some additional training since qualifying. They had been in their present posts from 2-23 years, but over two thirds had been in post for five years or less.

Caseload profiles

Health visitors were asked about their caseloads during 1987. The numbers of families with children under five on caseloads ranged from below 30 (for the health visitor who worked 10 hours a week) to over 300 families for some full-time health visitors. Numbers of children under five on a caseload ranged from 35 to over 400.

All health visitors had a number of Priority families. These are families that meet a range of criteria which are considered to put children at risk and therefore in need of closer health visitor contact. A list of criteria is used (see Appendix III) but a wide degree of discretion is allowed each health visitor regarding which families are recorded as a 'priority'. Once recorded as such, the health visitor is required to write a regular report and review the family with their Community Nurse Specialist. For some this additional work appeared to operate as a disincentive to register a family as a priority and so a two tier system operated; there were formally registered Priority families and those on whom health visitors informally kept a close eye. In addition, 15 of the 21 health visitors interviewed had some children under five who were on the social services' Child Protection Register in 1987.

In the group discussions, health visitors estimated that the number of failure to thrive children per caseload was between 2 and 3. When the 21 health visitors were interviewed about specific failure to thrive children on their caseloads, four could not recall any children under five who fell onto the 3rd centile in 1987, whilst others recalled between 1 and 6, giving a total sample of 39 children, and a mean figure of 1.85 per caseload.

Clinic attendance

Nearly half the 21 health visitors interviewed said they routinely visited families at home if they chose not to attend the child health clinics. In addition, it became apparent that health visitors would not expect to have much contact with children aged 2-5 years, except for the three year developmental check. Some health visitors commented that clinics had little to offer children or their parents at this stage of their development. Others saw mothers' groups (eg, run by social services) as a way of attracting those who made little use of child health clinics.

Access to weighing scales

A clear pre-requisite for health visitors to measure weight gain or loss is access to accurate weighing equipment. In the individual interviews, nine health visitors expressed satisfaction with access to scales. Several had their own set, or had what they described as "very easy access". However, ten were dissatisfied with weighing equipment. For some the problem was having no accurate scales; some health visitors stated that certain sets "weighed light". They said this raised few problems so long as they used the same set every time to weigh a particular child. However, it did present difficulties if they had to alternate between a set that "weighed light" and one that "weighed heavy". A frequent complaint was having to share sets with other health visitors, and having no good portable scales for home weighing. Two health visitors reported they had written to charities to obtain money to buy scales.

Communication channels with key professionals.

Health visitors were asked to rate on a four point scale the quality of channels of communication with key professional colleagues (Table 1).

TABLE 1

PERCENTAGE DISTRIBUTIONS OF HEALTH VISITOR RATINGS OF COMMUNICATION CHANNELS WITH KEY PROFESSIONALS

	GOOD %	ADEQUATE %	POOR %	NONE %	TOTAL %
GPs	48	33	14	5	100
CMOs	90	5	0	5	100
PAEDIATRICIANS	50	45	0	5	100
SOCIAL SERVICES	55	35	10	0	100
SUPERVISOR	45	50	5	0	100

It is noticeable that, apart from communication withClinical Medical Officers, only about half those interviewed reported good communication channels with key professionals. These findings could have important implications for the design of the referral process for any project for children failing to thrive. If referrals by health visitors were to be routed via general practitioners or paediatricians, then channels of communication would need to be improved.

Referral of failure to thrive children

Health visitors were clear about courses of action open to them should a child be failing to thrive. Once a child dropped below the 3rd centile for weight they could refer to the paediatrician, via the GP or Clinical Medical Officer. Sometimes they chose not to refer, eg, when they were sure the child was failing to gain weight as the mother was continuing to breast feed when she had insufficient milk. In their experience such children thrived once they went on to solids. At other times health visitors found their referral blocked by a GP or Clinical Medical Officer who did not share their concern.

Health visitors expressed frustration when referral to the paediatrician did not 'cure' the failure to thrive. Some complained that all the paediatricians did was review the child at the outpatient clinic every six months. Others reported that, in such situations, "all the paediatricians do is tell the health visitors to monitor". When health visitors were requested to keep a check on a child's weight (eg, by a paediatrician or social worker), low clinic attendance by some families meant this request could not always be fulfilled. Health visitors have no legal sanctions to ensure attendance. In the few cases where a child was the subject of a Care Order or Supervision Order, they reported this sometimes improved attendance at clinics for weighing.

Concerns were expressed in the group discussions about children under five who were developmentally delayed. Health visitors estimated that for every child below the 3rd centile there were about three children who were above the 3rd centile but below the 10th, and were developmentally delayed. These children were (in the health visitors' opinions) understimulated as a result of social or emotional deprivation. They would constantly be referred for developmental checks and rechecks, but were never quite 'bad enough' for any action by the paediatricians or by social services. As one health visitor said, "Sometimes you wish they would drop below the 3rd centile so you could refer them". It was clear that these children created much anxiety for health visitors.

Three referral routes were available to health visitors for developmentally delayed children. These were priority day care, Opportunity Groups and the Child and Family Guidance Service. The priority day care budget, funded by social services, offers day care where a family is at risk of breakdown for medical or social reasons. This service is provided to assist parents in fulfilling their parental role and to help a child realise her or his developmental potential. However, referral criteria had recently been tightened due to overspending of the budget, so access to priority day care had been reduced. The Opportunity Groups are for pre-school children with special needs. These range from children with specific handicaps (eg, Down's Syndrome) to social deprivation. The groups were experiencing a demand for places that was beyond their capacity. Consequently they were perceived by health visitors as less likely to take socially deprived or developmentally delayed children. Finally, a health visitor could refer the child, parent or family to the Child and Family Guidance Service or to a clinical psychologist, but for these services a lack of transport for some families was seen by health visitors to be a problem.

Additional resources for children failing to thrive and their families

Suggestions from the health visitor interviews fell into three groups. Firstly, half those interviewed suggested additional resources outside the home were needed. For example, support groups for mothers of failure to thrive children and centres to train parents in basic parenting and housekeeping skills were proposed. In the group discussions health visitors raised the issue of designing a service for failure to thrive children that would be acceptable to a range of families. They anticipated some parents would not make use of a 'family centre' type resource because of the stigma attached to attending such centres. There were also suggestions for specialised playgroups or nurseries that would not carry the stigma of Opportunity Groups. Secondly, one third of the health visitors argued for increased resources going into the homes of children failing to thrive. Suggestions included the appointment of more social services family aides and the recruitment of volunteers or experienced 'grannies', to teach home-making skills and stimulate children. Thirdly, a quarter of those interviewed wanted more time for health visitors to increase their input with failure to thrive children, in particular to observe actual feeding of the children by parents.

Data on children under five on or below the 3rd centile in 1987

From the interviews with the 21 health visitors, we obtained information on 39 children whose weight was on or below the 3rd centile at some point during 1987, and were under five at that time. There were 23 girls and 16 boys. For much of the following analysis we have expressed numbers as percentages, to make comparison easier. However, it should be remembered that the sample size is only 39.

Information on demographic features of the sample were collected from health visitors (see questionnaire in Appendix II). At the time of initial concern about the child's low weight, 67% of the children lived in a household in which at least one parent was in employment, 54% lived in council housing whilst 33% were owner-occupiers and 23% lived in single-parent households. Whilst the sample appeared to over-represent families in low socio-economic groups, it was not drawn exclusively from such groups. This accords with the literature that has established that failure to thrive children can be found across all socio-economic groups.

Nearly half of the sample (49%) was on the health visitors' Priority Lists although, as already discussed, some health visitors operated a two tier system, with a number of children on their own unofficial priority list. Eight of the 39 children (21%) had been on the social services Child Protection Register at some time.

Birth weights of children in the sample ranged from 1.4 kg to 3.85 kg, with a mean weight of 2.9 kg. Centile charts show that for a full-term birth the 50th centile weight is about 3.5 kg. Three children were known to have been premature babies and this was taken into account when their position on the centile charts was calculated. A quarter of the sample (26%) was below the 3rd centile at birth, whilst two thirds (66%) were on or above the 10th centile. However, the degree of weight deviation of these children can be gauged by the finding that, at the time of the health visitor interviews, only 36% of the sample were on or above the 10th centile whilst 38% were below the 3rd centile.

Health visitors were asked about the diagnosis of each child's failure to thrive. If the child had been hospitalised they usually had a discharge letter with the paediatrician's diagnosis. In other cases, the health visitors themselves were asked for their diagnosis. Three diagnostic categories emerged; these were non-organic, organic and 'small child'. The first two diagnostic categories are commonly used within the failure to thrive literature. The third is not unique to this study. Evidence to the panel conducting the inquiry into the death of Kimberley Carlile (Carlile 1987) suggested that she was a "small child", although the panel rejected this explanation, concluding that she "...should have never been regarded as a small child. She ought, moreover, never to have become a small child".

Two children had no diagnosis from the health visitor or paediatrician, 18 were diagnosed as non-organic, 11 as organic and 8 as 'small child'. The mean birth weight for the non-organic and 'small' categories was 3.1 kg, which is close to the 10th centile, whereas the mean birth weight of those diagnosed as cases of organic failure to thrive was less than 2.4 kg and hence below the 3rd centile.

When we compared the demographic details of the 18 non-organic failure to thrive children with the other 21 children, then the following picture emerged. The group diagnosed as non-organic had a lower percentage of parents in employment (44% as compared to 86% for the other children) and a lower percentage of owner-occupiers (10% as compared to 52%). There was a higher percentage living in single-parent families (39% as compared to 10%). As a group they had also experienced more significant family changes (such as death, divorce, birth, unemployment or move of house) than the rest of the sample; on average 1.83 changes compared to 0.73 for the remainder. More of these children were described by health visitors as having been developmentally delayed at some stage (47% as compared to 29% for the remainder of the sample). All eight children in the sample who had been on the Child Protection Register and eight of the nine children described by health visitors as low clinic attenders were diagnosed as non-organic.

These findings are in direct contrast to the 8 children whose failure to thrive was explained in terms of being a 'small child'. None of these were developmentally delayed, nor were they low clinic attenders or on the Child Protection Register. Of the 8 diagnosed as 'small child', 6 lived in two-parent households where at least one parent was in employment. It may be that factors such as these are used by health professionals in deciding whether to diagnose as non-organic or as 'small', once an organic base has been excluded. Only one of the children diagnosed as 'small' could be described as having been small at birth, with a birth centile below the 3rd; seven were on or above the 10th centile at birth. Thus the diagnosis of 'small' seems to rest on the absence of factors associated with deprivation, rather than on positive evidence of a child being constitutionally small.

Children's weight patterns between the time concern was first expressed and the time of the health visitor interviews were examined. We had hypothesised that children might follow one of three patterns; 'constants', 'divers' and 'dippers'. We found that the children in our sample could be categorised in this way. A 'constant' pattern was followed by 28%, staying below the 3rd centile. A further 28% fitted the pattern of 'dippers', crossing and recrossing the 3rd centile on more than one occasion. The third group (44%) broadly followed the pattern of 'divers'; that is, at the time of the research interviews, they had climbed back above the 3rd centile, having previously dived below it. However, our hypotheses regarding the reasons for these patterns were only partly supported by the data. For example, we hypothesised that the 'divers' would be suffering from organic failure to thrive, but this was only the diagnosis for 5 of the 17 children who followed this weight pattern. Centile charts for height were too rarely completed to determine if the 11 'constants' were stunted in all-round growth, but 4 of them had been diagnosed as 'small', suggesting their overall growth might have been below the norm for their age. Finally, we hypothesised the 11 'dippers' might have suffered several short-term organic conditions and/or non-organic episodes of failure to thrive associated with family stress. Regular intervention (eg, hospital, or intensive health visitor input) would have ensured such children climbed above the 3rd centile, only to drop below it once the intervention ceased. We found that for 7 of these children there were recurrent episodes of illness, short hospital admissions, feeding problems and/or periods of family stress that necessitated the involvement of health or social services staff.

So far our discussion has centered around the diagnoses of failure to thrive, and the patterns of weight loss and gain. However, we were also interested in the outcome of children's failure to thrive episode(s), and so we divided them into Improvers and Non-Improvers. The children who followed the patterns of 'constants' and 'dippers' were categorised as Non-Improvers, since they were either constantly below the 3rd centile or had had successive episodes of low weight. The 'divers' were categorised as Improvers, regarding the outcome of their failure to thrive, since they had now established a weight above the 3rd centile after only one episode below it. This gave us 17

Improvers and 22 Non-Improvers. Initially we examined the demographic factors of the two categories to see if there were any features that distinguished the Improvers from the Non-Improvers. However, we found there were no strong distinguishing factors between them in terms of, for example, parents' unemployment (29% compared to 36%) or single-parent households (24% compared to 23%).

We then examined the outcome categories by diagnosis, as we were interested in whether diagnosis was a useful predictor of outcome (Table 2).

TABLE 2

PERCENTAGE DISTRIBUTIONS OF OUTCOMES BY DIAGNOSIS OF FAILURE TO THRIVE

	ORGANIC	NON-ORGANIC	NOT DIAGNOSED/ 'SMALL'
	(N=11)	(N=18)	(N=10)
	%	%	%
IMPROVERS	45	44	40
NON-IMPROVERS	55	56	60
TOTAL	100	100	100

From Table 2 it can be seen that outcomes were similarly distributed across the three diagnoses of organic, non-organic, and the not diagnosed/ 'small' children. Across the categories, between 40% and 45% had improved whilst from 55% to 60% had not, suggesting that diagnosis bore little or no relationship to outcome.

However, the one factor that did distinguish between the Improvers and the Non-Improvers was whether they had been hospitalised, and if so, whether they gained weight in hospital or not. At this stage this was a tentative conclusion, since only 20 of the 39 children had been into hospital. These 20 comprised 41% of the Improvers, whilst 60% of the Non-Improvers were admitted, as shown in Table 3.

TABLE 3

PERCENTAGE DISTRIBUTION OF HOSPITAL ADMISSION FOR FAILURE TO THRIVE INVESTIGATION BY OUTCOME

	IMPROVER (N=17)	NON-IMPROVER (N=22)
	%	%
HOSPITAL ADMISSION	41	60
NO ADMISSION	59	40
TOTAL	100	100

Information on weight loss or gain in hospital was only available on 10 of the 20 hospitalised children (Table 4). Of the 4 hospitalised Improvers, 3 lost weight in hospital and 1 gained. This compared with the 6 Non-Improvers, all of whom gained weight when in hospital.

TABLE 4

DISTRIBUTION OF OUTCOMES BY WEIGHT CHANGE IN HOSPITAL, FOR THOSE ADMITTED FOR FAILURE TO THRIVE INVESTIGATIONS

N=20

	WEIGHT GAIN	WEIGHT LOSS	WEIGHT N/K	TOTAL
IMPROVERS	1	3	3	7
NON-IMPROVERS	6	0	7	13
TOTAL	7	3	10	20

Table 3 shows that the Non-Improvers were more likely to have been admitted to hospital than the Improvers. Table 4 shows they were also more likely to have gained weight whilst there. Yet their outcome as Non-Improvers suggests this weight gain was to no avail.

Most children on admission to hospital for medical reasons initially lose weight (Jones et al 1987). If Improvers are more likely to lose weight when in hospital then they are following this pattern. For weight-losers it may be that the hospital feeding regime is not as good at meeting the child's needs as that the child experiences at home; this, combined with the stress of being away from home, could account for the loss.

If Non-Improvers were more likely to gain weight in hospital, then one explanation might be that the hospital feeding regime was better at meeting the child's needs than that which the child experienced at home. Perversely, weight gain in hospital might also, for some children, contribute to future weight loss. Having a child who failed to thrive at home, but who thrives in hospital, may further reduce a parent's sense of competence, compound feelings of inadequacy or guilt, and so make weight gain after discharge even less likely.

These tentative conclusions fit with the findings in some of the child abuse enquiries, in which children have gained weight in a setting away from home and then lost it on their return (Beckford 1985; Carlile 1987). They also fit with the literature regarding the importance of feeding interaction for children failing to thrive, and the part feeding problems can play in the ongoing problem.

From these findings we hypothesised that presence or absence of feeding problems would be related to outcome, with children who exhibited such problems being least likely to have improved with regard to their failure to thrive. To test this hypothesis we re-examined our original data for any details of feeding difficulties parents or others had reported in relation to the failure to thrive children. The questionnaire (Appendix II) had not included a question specifically relating to feeding difficulties. However, for 21 of the 39 children, health visitors had made reference to feeding problems in the course of describing the child's failure to thrive (Table 5). These were usually the health visitors' own comments, or the reported comments of the children's mothers. Some references to feeding problems were included in the paediatrician's correspondence. Examples were the mothers being reported as saying the children had small appetites, or were poor, fussy or reluctant feeders. One health visitor described a child as refusing to eat, whilst another said one baby was "never interested in feeding".

TABLE 5

PERCENTAGE DISTRIBUTIONS OF OUTCOMES BY PRESENCE OR ABSENCE OF FEEDING PROBLEMS

	FEEDING PROBLEMS NOTED (N=21) %	NO FEEDING PROBLEMS NOTED (N=18) %
IMPROVERS	29	61
NON-IMPROVERS	71	39
TOTAL	100	100

Of those children for whom feeding problems had been noted by their health visitor, 71% did not improve. By contrast, of those for whom no reference to feeding problems was made by the health visitor only 39% did not improve. These findings support our hypothesis that feeding problems are related to the failure to thrive outcome.

4. CONCLUSIONS FROM THE FIRST STUDY

In conclusion, our discussions and interviews with health visitors suggest that children below the 3rd centile cause concern. Clear avenues for referral to paediatricians exist, but on occasions some children are sent back for the health visitor to monitor weight change. Such children are a particular source of worry for health visitors since they have not been 'cured', and health visitors usually have no other avenues of referral or means of intervention available to them. Another group of children who create anxiety for health visitors are those between the 3rd and 10th centile, who are seen to be suffering from social or emotional deprivation. In terms of their opportunities to refer children then clearly it was this group that made them feel as if they were 'left holding the baby', perhaps literally as well as metaphorically. Health visitors have no resources for such children, unless the situation is sufficiently severe to warrant intervention by social workers. High health visitor turnover, a wide net for determining Priority cases, lack of adequate administrative support and concern over the adequacy of weighing equipment must enhance feelings of pressure.

Precise knowledge of children's centile lines was often not available to health visitors, since much of the weighing equipment they used was reported to be inadequate or inaccurate. Weighing of children is an activity that is central to surveillance of children's health and development. The poor quality of equipment was recognised to be a problem, but action to improve the situation seemed to rest with individuals, and had a variable success rate. Some health visitors seemed resigned to having equipment that was inadequate. We found this surprising in view of the emphasis now placed on completing centile charts for all children from birth, the evidence on the long-term effects of failure to thrive and its value as an indicator of social and medical problems. One view expressed to us was that weighing was undertaken primarily as a means of building relationships with parents, rather than as an end in itself. This might account for health visitors' apparent resignation to this state of affairs.

From the data on children below the 3rd centile, it was clear that those diagnosed as non-organic failure to thrive possessed a range of factors not present in those diagnosed as organic or 'small'. Basically, the factors present in the non-organic group were those commonly associated with poverty. We gained an impression that non-organic failure to thrive was often diagnosed when paediatricians were unable to find an organic cause. Children were diagnosed as 'small' when no organic basis for their failure to thrive could be found and factors associated with poverty were not present.

However, we then looked at outcome as well as diagnosis. We re-examined the data by comparing those children who were gaining weight with those who were staying the same or losing weight. Two factors of significance emerged. The first was the link between outcome and weight gain or loss in hospital. Most children initially lose weight on admission to hospital. If children who were failing to thrive gained weight in hospital, only to fail to sustain the rate of gain after discharge, this suggests feeding is a substantive issue, even if not the original cause of the failure to thrive. Therefore we re-examined our data for information on feeding difficulties. We found that those children who appeared to be getting better were significantly less likely to have had feeding problems identified by health visitors.

These findings were based on a very small number of cases. However, when taken together with the literature review, they led us to the conclusion that there was a need to explore feeding problems as the pivotal issue which divided those children who improved from those who remained below the 3rd centile, or who crossed and recrossed it. On the basis of the findings from this first study we decided to undertake a second study focusing more closely on feeding problems and looking in more detail at children's weight patterns since birth. In designing the second study it was also possible to address some of the limitations of the first study's research design.

Section 3

The Second Study

1. THE RESEARCH DESIGN AND PROCESS FOR THE SECOND STUDY

The sample for Study 2 was based on the same geographical area as the first, but used the caseloads of the 30 health visitors in the area who had not been interviewed in Study 1. For the majority of these caseloads, there had been a change of health visitor over the past 18 months. In the first study we had relied on health visitors' recall to identify children on or below the 3rd centile. In this second study we did not interview health visitors but examined their clinic cards and, for some children, health visitor records to identify those who had been on or below the 3rd centile in the study period. We checked children's weights against the current centile chart used by the district health authority. At this stage of screening caseloads, a note was made of any child who appeared to be on or below the 3rd centile in 1987. In total we examined some 6-8,000 clinic cards as well as about 2,000 health visitor records.

Once children on or below the 3rd centile had been identified, we studied in more detail the clinic cards and health visitor notes relating to those children. We recorded each child's weight at birth and one weeks gestation and all subsequent weights and ages. If it was made clear in the clinic card whether the child had been weighed clothed or naked, this was also noted. A standard allowance of 1 lb, or 0.45 kg, was deducted from clothed weights before the weight was plotted on the centile chart. We also recorded any references in the clinic card or health visitor notes to feeding problems, up to and including the time when the child was below the 3rd centile. In addition, information on hospital admissions (including to special care baby units), and weight loss or gain whilst in hospital for failure to thrive investigations was extracted. For this study we decided against gathering demographic data on the children in the sample. Our findings in Study 1 showed little or no relationship between demographic factors and outcome, although a close association between demographic factors and diagnosis existed.

Paediatric notes on all children in the sample who had been admitted to the district hospital were also examined. Their weight loss or gain in hospital was noted, plus any data relating to the child's feeding difficulties and parent-child interaction around feeding. In the course of gathering data it became clear that although all children lived within one health district, some had been admitted to neighbouring hospitals in other health districts as in-patients. We did not have access to the records of these hospitals.

Initial screening of the 30 health visitor caseloads gave a preliminary list of 121 children who appeared to fit the study criteria. Of the children on this initial list, 20 were excluded at the stage of data extraction. Due to difficulties in reading the information on some of the charts, when we looked more closely at the notes the weights of 7 of the children were found to be above the 3rd centile. A total of 11 children were on or below the 3rd centile in 1986 and/or 1988, but no recorded weights could be found for 1987. Finally, 2 children were excluded as their families were only briefly resident in the area, and hence their health records were too scant to build up any picture of their progress. This gave a sample of 101 children across 30 health visitor caseloads.

On the basis of our research findings from Study 1 and the literature we had examined, we refined our definitions of Improver and Non-Improver for use in analysis of data in Study 2. In particular we wanted to take into account the length of time the child had been below the 3rd centile. We concluded that any child who had spent less than six months below the 3rd centile and who had then regained a previously established weight pattern, we would categorise as an Improver. Any child who had been below the 3rd centile for ten months or more, even if they had then established a higher weight, and any child that had repeatedly dipped across the 3rd centile, no matter what their most recent weight centile position, we would categorise as a Non-Improver. Since the literature on the effects of malnutrition was not specific about how long 'too long' below the 3rd centile was, we decided that any children who had dipped below the 3rd centile for 6-9 months, and re-established a weight above the 3rd should be categorised as Borderline.

2. FINDINGS FROM STUDY 2

Our initial task in this study was to identify from the clinic records all children at or below the 3rd centile. As our investigations progressed it became clear that the way in which information was recorded was having a considerable influence on what should have been a simple, if somewhat laborious, task. Therefore, we comment on issues relating to the way records are kept as well as analysing the data we extracted from them. In making these observations we are aware that the majority of our sample in Study 2 was drawn from caseloads where there had been a change of health visitor. We do not feel this invalidates our comments since health visitor turnover affects every caseload at some point.

Health visitor records and clinic cards

The health visitor notes and entries in the child health clinic cards we examined were handwritten. In some instances this caused problems of legibility. Records were concise because the space available limits the amount that may be written. Some health visitors overcame this limitation by tiny writing or folding copies of correspondence very small. There is a high level of duplication between health visitor records and clinic cards. Storage of records was also a problem. Some filing systems were so overcrowded that it was impossible to find notes without removing half the contents.

A major problem in extracting data for the study was that recorded weights frequently vacillated between imperial and metric scales. In addition, the scale being used was not always made explicit; for example, an entry of '7.2' could mean 7 pounds 2 ounces or 7.2 kilogrammes. Health visitors did not always specify whether a child had been weighed clothed or naked. This could make a considerable difference in a child's position on a growth assessment chart. Some children were in plaster or a removable splint for correction of a hip displacement. Whether or not the child was in the plaster or splint at the time of weighing was rarely made clear in health visitor or paediatric records.

Older versions of the centile charts were printed on paper and although too large for health records they could easily be folded. The new charts in use were printed on thin card. They are still larger than the health visitor notes so are folded; this makes some charts illegible around the line of the fold.

These charts are also taller than the paper envelopes used in some of the clinics to hold children's clinic cards and already many looked dog- eared.

Some children had no centile chart in their notes. We assume this is due to the fact that charts have only recently been made widely available in the health district. For children who did have charts in their notes, these were often incomplete or inaccurate. It was also common to find two charts in one child's record card; frequently one was completely blank. The largest number of charts found in any one child's notes was four. In this instance, each chart had only a few weights entered, so no overall picture of the child's growth could be obtained until all the weights had been entered onto one chart. However, the picture was somewhat different for the youngest children in the study; generally they had one centile chart completed from birth.

We plotted weights for all the sample onto charts, joining the entries with a straight line to estimate each child's growth pattern between weights. Whilst this is unlikely to give a totally accurate picture it is the procedure used by health visitors. The match between actual and estimated weight gain is closest when the child is weighed frequently. The longer the gaps between weights, the greater the chance that the child's actual weight deviates from the line plotted on the chart. Whilst this was rarely a problem for children under 6 months, after this age it was not unusual to find a 6-12 month gap between recorded weights. In general, health visitor contact with children declines as they grow older, so they are weighed less frequently. In some cases this resulted in long gaps between a child's first recorded weight below the 3rd centile and their next weight check. In such cases it might be that the low weight gain was not recognised or, if recognised, was either not a cause for concern or the concern was not acted upon.

As we progressed with the data collection it became apparent that there existed on health visitors' caseloads many unrecognised low weight-gaining children. For example, an 18 month old child was weighed by the clinical medical officer at a developmental assessment. "Healthy" was all that was written on the child's card, despite the fact that her weight was on that occasion below the 3rd centile and she had crossed three major centile lines since birth. No reassessment was arranged and so the child was not weighed again until her three year developmental assessment, when she was still below the 3rd centile. Another child had been below the 3rd centile for about a year before it was recognised. In this case, once the low weight had been identified, six-month follow-ups were arranged. By the time of the first follow-up the child had regained its position above the 10th centile, as it had been after birth. Had selection of the sample relied on health visitor recall, as it had in the first study, it seems likely that such children would not have been identified. Finally, one child was initially recognised as a low weight gainer by the health visitor, but action was left to its parents who were themselves members of the medical profession. Thus, so far as the primary health care team was concerned, the child's subsequent weight status went unrecognised since it was unknown to them.

Paediatric records

There were paediatric records on almost half the children in the sample. Two were empty folders, just with the child's admission number recorded on it. The remainder contained notes on children's admissions to the paediatric ward or the special care baby unit and copies of correspondence regarding out- patient appointments. We sought information on weight loss or gain for those children who were in-patients for failure to thrive, as well as any out-patient weights to supplement the data on the children's centile charts.

Children's weights on admission to hospital were easy to locate but weights on discharge were not. Even amongst the children who had been admitted for failure to thrive there was one for whom we could not find a discharge weight recorded in the notes. Some children had weight centile charts but, as with those in the health visitor notes, not all were completed. One child had several hospital admissions for bilateral hip dislocation that required surgery. The child was regularly weighed as part of the hospital admission procedure, as well as by the health visitor, but no recognition of failing growth was apparent from the records. The paediatric notes contained three centile charts; two had only one weight entered and the third was completely blank. When all the available weights were plotted it was clear that the child had been below the 3rd centile for nearly 2 years.

Children on or below the 3rd centile in 1987

There were 101 children in the sample; 57 girls and 44 boys. Birth weights ranged from 0.98 kg to 4.1 kg, with a mean weight of 2.91 kg. This is almost identical to the mean birth weight in Study 1 (2.9 kg).

In Study 1 only 8% of the sample had been premature, whilst in this second study the percentage of premature births was 20%. This may be due to some health visitors in the first study not viewing premature babies as part of the failure to thrive population and so not recalling such children. Prematurity was taken into account when weights were plotted on centile charts. Five of the 21 premature infants had a birth weight on or below the 3rd centile but they all achieved a weight above the 3rd centile within the first few months of life. The mean birth weight of the 80 full-term infants in the sample was 3.1 kg, which is close to the 10th centile.

Although we started with a sample of 101 children, we excluded 12 from the main data analysis. As already discussed, deviation from a previously established weight pattern is widely used as the means to identify children who are not thriving, and therefore at risk of impaired or delayed development. Thus we excluded from our sample 9 children who were born below the 3rd centile and had remained at or below it, never establishing a weight pattern above the 3rd. Such children have never demonstrated that they have the capacity to achieve a higher weight-for-age. Their slow growth may be the result of limited genetic potential, due to having small parents or because of intra-uterine problems that result in impairment of the child's capacity for growth and development in all spheres. A further 3 children in the sample suffered from specific syndromes that are known to result in stunted growth. Even under optimum feeding conditions they may never have achieved normal growth. We decided to exclude them although we acknowledge that such children's growth potential, limited as it is, might be further checked by feeding difficulties. Therefore, the final sample we analysed comprised a total of 89 children.

We initially categorised the 89 children according to their weight pattern from birth up to their last recorded weight into 'constants', 'dippers' and 'divers'. As in Study 1 we then collapsed these categories by outcome. The sample was divided into Improvers (less than 6 months below the 3rd centile), Non-Improvers (below the 3rd centile for 10 months or more, or repeated dips below the 3rd) and Borderline. Included amongst the Borderline category were children who were weighed so infrequently that we could only estimate that they were below the 3rd centile for about 6-9 months.

The distribution of cases by birth centile and outcome is shown in Table 6. Two thirds (61) were categorised as Non-Improvers, 17 as Improvers and 11 as Borderline.

TABLE 6

DISTRIBUTION OF CASES BY BIRTH CENTILE AND OUTCOME

N=89

OUTCOME: BIRTH CENTILE:	IMPROVERS	NON-IMPROVERS	BORDERLINE	TOTAL
AT< 3RD	2	9	4	15
3RD < 10TH	3	21	1	25
10TH < 50TH	7	27	3	37
ABOVE 50TH	5	4	3	12
TOTAL	17	61	11	89

As can be seen in Table 6, 40 of the final sample had a birth weight below the 10th centile whilst only 12 were above the 50th. However, when birth centile is examined in relation to outcome category, less than a third of the Improvers had a birth weight below the 10th centile, whilst over a quarter were above the 50th. Non-Improvers accounted for the highest proportion of low birth weight children, with half below the 10th centile.

In Study 1, one factor that had distinguished between Improvers and Non-Improvers was whether or not they had been hospitalised for investigation of their failure to thrive, and whether they had gained or lost weight whilst in hospital. In Study 2, of the 89 children in the final sample, only 9 had been admitted to hospital for failure to thrive investigations (see Table 7). When admissions are examined by outcome category, the differences are small, with 6% of the Improvers admitted, and 11% of the combined Non-Improvers and Borderline. Of those admitted, 2 had gone to hospitals outside the district

45

health authority and no data on weight loss or gain were available. Of the remaining 7, all gained weight in hospital.

TABLE 7

OUTCOME CATEGORY BY HOSPITAL TREATMENT/ INVESTIGATION FOR FAILURE TO THRIVE, CONTROLLING FOR WEIGHT CHANGE IN HOSPITAL

N=89

	HOSPITAL ADMISSION WEIGHT NOT KNOWN	HOSPITAL ADMISSION WEIGHT UP	NO HOSPITAL ADMISSION
IMPROVERS	0	1	16
NON-IMPROVERS	1	5	55
BORDERLINE	1	1	9
TOTAL	2	7	80

For only one child whose weight went up in hospital was the rate of gain sustained on discharge to the extent of taking the child into the Improver category. The health visitor's notes on this breast-fed baby referred to advice given to the mother to give the baby top-up bottle feeds. This advice was not acted upon until reiterated by the paediatrician after the child had been admitted to hospital. Thus for this child it appeared that the hospital admission resulted in a successful intervention around feeding problems.

Another factor in which we were interested was whether prematurity or time in a special care baby unit (SCBU) divided children whom we categorised as Improvers from those categorised as Non-Improvers (Table 8). In the final sample of 89 children, 22 had been premature births, and/or had been in the special care baby unit. Such a high figure is not surprising as the association between tube feeding (often necessary for babies in special care units), lack of a vigorous sucking reflex (found in some premature babies) and subsequent poor weight gain has been well documented in the literature.

TABLE 8

OUTCOME CATEGORY BY PREMATURITY/SPECIAL CARE
BABY UNIT (SCBU)

N=89

	PREMATURE PLUS SCBU	SCBU ONLY	PREMATURE ONLY	NOTPREM NOT SCBU
IMPROVERS	2	2	0	13
NON-IMPROVERS	7	0	9	45
BORDERLINE	0	0	2	9
TOTAL	9	2	11	67

Of the 61 Non-Improvers in the sample, a total of 16 (26%) were premature and/or in SCBU. The percentage figure was broadly similar for the Improvers and the Borderline cases (24% and 18%). Thus, whilst being premature or in SCBU puts children at risk of low weight gain at some stage, it is not an indicator of longer term outcome, as defined in this study.

Our hypothesis from Study 1 was that presence or absence of feeding problems would be related to children's outcome category. In Study 2 we paid particular attention at the stage of data collection to any information relating to such problems. Our first analysis was to count all references to feeding problems in the records held by health visitors. We found the number of problems for the 89 children ranged from 0-8, with the mean number of problems being 2.02. For the 61 children categorised as Non- Improvers, 44% had three or more feeding problems recorded, as compared to only 9% of the Borderline category and 12% of the Improvers. However, we also found that for 23 of the 89 children, no feeding problems whatsoever were recorded in their notes, and this number included 14 of the 61 children categorised as Non-Improvers. This ran contrary to our hypothesis and so we decided to re-examine our data.

We already knew, from the data collection stage of the study, that there were children in the sample whose low weight had apparently passed unrecognised. Therefore at this stage of the analysis we divided the sample into recognised and unrecognised slow weight gainers and/or weight losers. Cases were classed as recognised if there were any comments on the clinic cards that demonstrated this (such as "onto 3rd centile" or "poor weight gain; to weigh monthly") or if they were referred to another health professional for investigation of their low weight gain. Cases were classed as unrecognised if there were no such comments in the notes and the children had not been referred to a clinical medical officer or paediatrician for investigations regarding their weight. In the sample of 89, 57 were classed as recognised low weight gainers, and 32 as unrecognised.

Having analysed the data in this way we then re-examined the distribution of feeding problems across the outcome categories. This time a clear picture emerged regarding the relationship between number of feeding problems and outcome, as is shown in Table 9.

Children recognised as low weight gainers and categorised as Improvers only averaged 1.4 recorded feeding problems. By contrast, those children who were recognised as low weight gainers and categorised as Non-Improvers averaged 3.2 recorded feeding problems. The Borderline with recognised low weight gain fell between the two, with an average of 1.7 feeding problems. Children whose low weight passed unrecognised had very few feeding problems recorded, irrespective of their outcome category.

Finally data on children who were premature or had been admitted to Special Care Baby Units were re-examined in relation to recognised and unrecognised low weight gainers (Table 10).

Of the 22 children who were premature and/or in SCBU, 77% were recognised as poor weight gainers, compared to 60% of the remainder of the sample being recognised as such. It may be that children who were premature and/or in SCBU are under close scrutiny at all times by health visitors, and so weight deviations are more likely to be picked up. Alternatively, having had a difficult or untimely start to their lives, parents may be more likely to report to health visitors any feeding difficulties or deviations in weight.

TABLE 9

OUTCOME CATEGORY BY MEAN NUMBER OF FEEDING PROBLEMS CONTROLLING FOR RECOGNISED OR UNRECOGNISED LOW WEIGHT GAIN

N=89

	LOW WEIGHT RECOGNISED		LOW WEIGHT UNRECOGNISED	
	NO. OF CASES	MEAN NO. OF FEEDING PROBS	NO. OF CASES	MEAN NO. OF FEEDING PROBS
CATEGORY:				
IMPROVERS	10	1.4	7	0.6
NON-IMPROVERS	41	3.2	20	0.9
BORDERLINE	6	1.7	5	0.8
TOTAL	57		32	

TABLE 10

PERCENTAGE DISTRIBUTIONS OF PREMATURITY/ADMISSION TO SPECIAL CARE BABY UNIT BY RECOGNITION OF LOW WEIGHT STATUS

	SCBU AND/OR PREMATURE (N=22) %	NOT SCBU NOT PREM (N=67) %
LOW WEIGHT STATUS:		
RECOGNISED	77	60
UNRECOGNISED	23	40
TOTAL	100	100

by health visitors, and so weight deviations are more likely to be picked up. Alternatively, having had a difficult or untimely start to their lives, parents may be more likely to report to health visitors any feeding difficulties or deviations in weight.

3. CONCLUSIONS FROM STUDY 2

In Study 1 we drew attention to the drawbacks of a research design that rested on health visitors' recall of children that fitted the research criteria. However, we hypothesised that for various reasons the level of recall would be quite high, although possibly biased towards younger children. This was upheld in Study 2, in which we found that the mean number of recognised low weight children per caseload was 1.9. This compares closely to the figure of 1.86 per caseload from health visitor recall in Study 1. From this we conclude that health visitors' recall of low weight children is good, once the low weight has been recognised.

This issue of recognition of low weight children loomed large in Study 2. For every two children recognised as low weight gainers, one child's low weight passed unrecognised. It appeared to us that, with one or two notable exceptions, completion or updating of centile charts was not a priority except where the health visitor had already identified a concern about the child's weight. Weight may be increasing whilst the rate of gain is dropping, but this would only be evident if the weights were plotted onto a centile chart. The charts did not seem to be used as a tool to help identify children whose weight gain was dropping off, but instead were used as evidence in support of an existing concern. This issue of acknowledging and acting on low weight has been highlighted in at least two child abuse inquiry reports. Firstly, the inquiry report following the death of Kimberley Carlile notes (Carlile 1987):

It was one cardinal feature of the failure in standards of care as provided for Kimberley that such [centile] charts were not properly used in her case. Had they been used and interpreted properly, the outcome for this ill-fated child might so easily have been different (p39).

Secondly, the report into the circumstances surrounding the death of Jasmine Beckford (Beckford 1985) states:

We conclude that, while Jasmine's weight did not go entirely unnoticed.....it was never properly taken on board by the doctors or the health visitors, and never at all by the social workers (p74).

We could say the same for the unrecognised low weight gainers in our study. Their weight did not go entirely unnoticed since they were weighed and their weights were recorded; this was the means by which we identified them. However, the low weight was never taken on board, in that it was not recognised as being of significance.

It was clear that the exploration and recording of feeding problems were related to health visitors' recognition of a child's low weight status, these children having a significantly higher number of feeding problems recorded. This suggests that once there is concern about a child's weight then possible reasons for it are explored. However, the mean number of feeding problems amongst the recognised low weight gainers (shown earlier in Table 9) also supported our hypothesis regarding the relationship between feeding problems and outcome. Children in this group who do not improve have more feeding problems than those who do. This has clear implications for the treatment of children who are failing to thrive.

Section 4

Treatment interventions

1. THE TREATMENT LITERATURE

It is important to state two substantive ways in which the treatment literature differs from our own work. Firstly, it is predominately based on the study of children who have been admitted to hospital, although this only comprises a very small part of the failure to thrive population. Secondly, it still often divides failure to thrive by the traditional organic and non- organic diagnoses.

A consequence of this is that much of the literature, in attempting to describe the causes of non-organic failure to thrive, is instead describing the causes of diagnosis. For example, Moore (1982) decribes failure to thrive in terms of, "The mother is usually depressed... Frequently, the failure to thrive baby is born into a single-parent family". In Study 1 we found that such factors only correlated with the diagnosis of non-organic failure to thrive. It did not act as a predictor of which children would improve and gain weight. We argued that diagnosis was in effect describing deprived children for whom no organic explanation of failure to thrive could be found. Therefore, in failing to make a discrimination based on outcome, the literature only describes the cause of the diagnosis, not the cause of failure to thrive.

But if these studies fail to identify the causes of failure to thrive why do so many have successful outcomes to their treatment programmes? There are two possible reasons. Firstly, whilst the literature describes a wide range of possible causes, the treatment proscribed mainly ignores these and instead concentrates on improving mother-child interaction around feeding. Secondly, by selecting for treatment on the basis of diagnosis (ie, those diagnosed as cases of non-organic failure to thrive) rather than on predicted outcome, the treatment commences with a head start. Not only does it include those for whom a poor or non-improving outcome to their failure to thrive is likely if no treatment is provided, but it also includes those who will improve without any treatment intervention.

With these limitations in mind, what does the literature tell us? Firstly, several studies comment on the prevalence of feeding problems amongst failure to thrive children. For example, Lachenmeyer and Davidovicz (1987), in their review article, cite studies that found differences in eating behaviour between failure to thrive children and children developing normally. They also referred to problems amongst failure to thrive children such as less vigorous sucking, which may result from prematurity or neurodevelopmental difficulties. Iwaniec et al (1985) studied 17 failure to thrive infants, comparing them with two contrast groups. All parents in the failure to thrive group reported specific feeding difficulties in their children, such as an inability, reluctance or refusal to suck milk, crying whilst being fed, vomiting and diarrhoea. Most reported more acute difficulties after the introduction of solids, when the children refused food, suffered increased vomiting and diarrhoea, screamed, regurgitated and showed an inability to swallow and chew. Pollitt et al (1975) reported that, in comparison to the contrast groups in their studies, failure to thrive children were more likely to present disturbances in eating. Over 50% of the mothers in the index group reported having difficulties feeding their children during the first 12 months. Finally, disordered feeding interaction was found by Bithoney and Newberger (1987) to be one of the ten major variables associated with failure to thrive, on the basis of factor analysis of variables drawn from interviews with mothers of failure to thrive children and matched controls.

Feeding difficulties, in conjunction with inadequacy of nutrition, can create a vicious cycle, to which the child and its caregiver contribute (Skuse 1985). The existence of such a cycle can make determining causality difficult. Lachenmeyer and Davidovicz (1987) conclude that whilst a disturbed mother-child relationship may be associated with the failure to thrive syndrome, it could not be assumed that the quality of the relationship caused it. However, this lack of established causal links need not stand in the way of effective intervention, since what started the failure to thrive may not be what is currently keeping it going. It is clear that for many children who are failing to thrive it is problems around feeding that perpetuate that cycle, even if they do not precipitate it.

Some studies, whilst exploring different outcomes, provide evidence in support of our general findings. A study of the relative success of foster parent placement and hospital care noted that one of their indicators, weight gain, was "a limited measure of success and is probably a poor predictor of outcome after the child has returned home" (Karniski et al 1986).

Therefore, the conclusion we draw from the literature, as well as from our own work, is that whilst causation may be a matter of some dispute, there is recognition of a link between failure to thrive and feeding problems. However, there is disagreement about the location and emphasis of treatment. Haynes et al (1984) argue for exploring different interventions based on their hypothesis of different "types" of mothers in their failure to thrive sample. Chatoor et al (1985) also support a differential approach based on an age-based classification of feeding disorders. Bithoney and Newberger (1987) recommend that social, behavioural and maternal-child interaction assessments should be obtained routinely as part of the initial diagnostic assessment of any child admitted to hospital with possible failure to thrive. Any interactional problems between the caretaker and child could be addressed prior to, or instead of, admission. However, some paediatric texts still recommend addressing the issues of caretaker-child interaction only after feeding in hospital has achieved a weight gain. This suggests an acceptance that failure to thrive is the result of interaction between the child's organic disturbance, psychological make-up and environment (Goldson 1986) may not yet be widespread.

Making parents feel guilty about their child's condition does not help achieve improvement. A number of studies have addressed this issue, specifying the means by which they have created a context for change. For example, families may be involved in hospital treatment of their child from the outset, and be given all credit for any progress that the child makes (Hufton & Oates 1977). Intervention may be based on the premise that non-organic failure to thrive is not wilful neglect on the parents' part, but a symptom of family dysfunction (Moore 1982). In Moore's "Project Thrive", supportive therapy was provided to families throughout the time their child was in hospital and continued beyond hospital discharge. Lachenmeyer and Davidovicz (1987) suggest taking a position with parents that indicates that they did not cause the feeding problems, but that changes in their behaviour can now bring about changes in the child's behaviour.

In designing any treatment model for failure to thrive children the above issues need to be taken into account. Targeting of particular age groups of children is important, not only because of the long term effects of failure to thrive, but also because the treatment regime may need to be varied according to the age of the child. It is important to identify parents who could be resistant to intervention, and to understand their reasons for resistance so that such issues might be addressed. The adoption of a co-operative, involving and non-blaming stance towards parents is vital if treatment is to be accepted, and a climate for change created.

Finally, despite the bias inherent in several of the projects' treatment populations, a positive feature that emerges is the high level of success achieved by adopting a behavioural approach to the treatment of failure to thrive. The model we particularly favour is that described by Iwaniec in a number of publications (Iwaniec, Herbert & Sluckin 1988; Iwaniec, Herbert & McNeish 1985; Iwaniec 1987).

2. A TREATMENT MODEL

In proposing a treatment model we have drawn on our own work and the treatment literature to answer three key questions. What is the target population? What is the best treatment intervention for that population? What factors might inhibit change?

Targeting

Targeting of interventions is essential, given limited resources. It is important to ensure that resources are directed at those most in need and likely to gain maximum benefit. One of our initial tasks was to develop a set of indicators which could define the target population for a failure to thrive project. From our studies we argued against using existing diagnostic categories, since outcome of the failure to thrive episode was more useful as a means of targeting interventions on those most at risk.

On the basis of our findings we suggest a failure to thrive project should target interventions on children who fit the following criteria. Firstly, children should have been at or below the 3rd centile for 6 months or more, or have had more than one episode below the 3rd centile at any time excluding birth. Children who have had such long-lasting or recurrent episodes of failure to thrive are at risk of delayed or permanently impaired development. Secondly they should already have established their potential to thrive, having achieved a weight pattern above the 3rd centile in the past. Finally, they should be between 6 months and 3 years of age, since this is the population that health visitors can best monitor.

We suggest the referral process to a failure to thrive project should be an automatic one, with all children meeting the criteria being seen by project staff. Automatic referral is necessary if the targeting system is to work effectively. However, a large number of children might fall within such broad criteria, making it necessary to narrow the initial intake of a project. We suggest that, in addition to applying the criteria specified above, a project might give priority to children who gain weight in hospital, but continue to fail to thrive after discharge. It might not accept children diagnosed as suffering from specific growth-limiting syndromes. Finally, it could use presence or absence of feeding problems, as reported by the child's health visitor, as a means of prioritising referrals. In the treatment literature it is suggested that the following are useful indicators of persistent feeding problems (Iwaniec et al 1985b):

ON LIQUIDS. An inability, reluctance or refusal to suck; frequent falling asleep when being fed; crying while being fed; vomiting; stretching out; diarrhoea.

AT POINT OF CHANGE TO SOLIDS. Persistent refusal to take solids; increased vomiting and diarrhoea; persistent screaming.

ON SOLIDS. Appears disinterested in food or loses interest quickly; refuses to be fed by not opening mouth, turning away or spitting food out; plays with food during meals and eats very little; engages in distracting games instead of eating.

Having clear criteria for a project's target population does not remove the need for assessment by project workers of children referred. Assessment is necessary to ensure that referred children fit the criteria. There are likely to be referrals of children who cause anxiety to health or social services staff, but who do not fall within the target group and so need screening out. An assessment of a referred child, which includes observation of the child being fed by parents in the home setting, enables the failure to thrive to be viewed in the context of the family (Drotar et al 1985). It also enables project staff to ascertain that interventions centred on feeding are acceptable to parents. A project would need to establish at the very outset a clear policy with the health authority, and with social services, regarding what action might be taken if parents of a child who is failing to thrive refuse intervention by project staff. Finally, assessment ensures that the timing of intervention is appropriate. For example, the presence of a previously undiagnosed illness might indicate that medical treatment should take priority, making it appropriate for admission to the project to be rescheduled. This is not a return to the traditional model of intervention only being offered to children without an organic base to their failure to thrive. Rather, it is an acknowledgement that in some cases intervention cannot proceed until immediate medical problems have been resolved. On occasions the resolution of medical problems may also result in the resolution of feeding problems, rendering inclusion in the project unnecessary.

Intervention

Targeting and assessment should ensure that the focus is on children who have demonstrated a capacity to thrive, who are currently failing to thrive and who, with their care-givers, are caught in a cycle of feeding problems. We believe the aims of intervention, as proposed by Iwaniec, Herbert and Sluckin (1988), should be as follows:

> Resolve feeding difficulties and improve feeding style, ie, modify maternal behaviour and responses during the act of feeding (by means of counselling, modelling and carefully structured feeding situations).
>
> Deliberately, and in a planned and graduated fashion, create positive interactions and reduce negative interactions....... between mother and child. We would usually attempt to desensitize the child's anxiety and fear of the mother's feeding and other caregiving activities... (p235-236).

Although Iwaniec et al specify mother-child interaction, the target of change is more accurately defined as caregiver-child interaction.

We have given considerable thought to the form of intervention a project might offer to children failing to thrive and their families. In general the child's home should be the setting in which intervention takes place, with the worker helping to create an atmosphere in which change is possible from first contact. Acknowledging parents as experts on their own child, who can teach the project worker about the particular problems they are experiencing, is a good means of beginning to enhance the parents' sense of competence.

Intervention should be structured and concentrate on a change in feeding patterns and behaviour, using such techniques as behaviour modification. Weights need to be measured and charted throughout any project-participant contact, and at its conclusion. The length of intervention will vary and be determined by a stabilised weight gain and an observed improvement in feeding by the child. A period of follow-up reinforcement and monitoring needs to occur after intervention has ceased.

Factors that might inhibit change

The obtaining of accurate weights of young children by health visitors is crucial if a failure to thrive project is to receive appropriate referrals. Health surveillance is rendered meaningless if accurate weighing is not possible. All health visitors need easy access to accurate, portable weighing devices. Attention also needs to be given to the accurate recording of information on centile charts and to the storage of such information when recorded. The current system is clearly inadequate. If the issues regarding weighing and recording can be effectively resolved then the next area for change concerns speedy identification of children at or below the third centile. The project model that we have outlined would rely on health visitors or project staff being able to identify easily children who match the referral criteria.

If a child has undergone medical investigation of low weight, this may have resulted in a diagnosis of non-organic failure to thrive. Such a diagnosis needs to be handled very sensitively if undermining of parents is to be avoided. Their sense of guilt and responsibility for their child's condition can easily be heightened, making it difficult to involve them in treatment.

As a failure to thrive project is likely to lie at the interface of health and social services, without being the managerial responsibility of either, attention needs to be given to achieving effective inter-agency communication, with the support of both managerial and professional staff in both sectors. In particular, project staff need support from management in other agencies if they are to resist pressures to widen their referral criteria. Targeting does not exclude an extension of a project should more resources become available. However, any extension needs to be undertaken in the light of reappraisal of the project as it stands, and after new criteria have been developed.

Section 5

Conclusions

We have conducted two research studies in one district of a local authority social services department in the south of England, on children under five who were below the third centile for weight in 1987. The studies were commissioned by The Children's Society who wished to develop a project for children who were failing to thrive. The first study relied on health visitor recall to identify those children on their caseloads who were below the third centile. We then used health visitor records and clinic cards to gather information on each child's weight pattern, treatment, interventions and outcomes, in addition to family composition, housing, parent employment and major changes such as divorce, illness or move of house. We also interviewed the health visitors about their caseloads, access to weighing scales and resources for children failing to thrive. In the second study we examined clinic cards to identify children fitting the research criteria. We again gathered information on each child's weight pattern, treatment and interventions, paying particular attention to feeding problems.

We used our data from Study 1 to build an understanding of the process by which health professionals reach a diagnosis of failure to thrive. Our impression was that initially an organic explanation for low weight was sought. If no such explanation was found, then any evidence of deprivation resulted in a non-organic diagnosis. If there was no organic explanation, nor any evidence of deprivation, then the child tended to be diagnosed as 'small'.

The demographic data collected in Study 1 indicated that the children came from across the whole socio-economic spectrum, a finding borne out by many other studies of children who fail to thrive. However, the data also suggested children diagnosed as 'small' were likely to be from two-parent, home-owning households with at least one parent in employment, in stark contrast to those diagnosed as cases of non-organic failure to thrive. This suggests that non-organic failure to thrive was a descriptive title for children living in deprivation, rather than a diagnosis. It was easy to see how non-organic failure to thrive was understood by some health visitors to be synonymous with deprivation.

Interviews with health visitors revealed their concerns that paediatricians did not always 'cure' failure to thrive children. Children without an organic condition were often passed back to health visitors, who had no other means of treatment or intervention available to them. Particular worries arose regarding children who were just above the third centile but who were, by the health visitors' assessments, understimulated as a result of social or emotional deprivation.

Had our analysis ended at this point, these findings could easily have led us to the conclusion that we needed to concentrate on issues related to poverty. From this we might have recommended that the needs of children failing to thrive would best be met by the provision of a 'family centre' resource, offering compensatory care to deprived children. However, when we went on to analyse failure to thrive in terms of outcome, the need for a different classification became apparent. In terms of who is likely to re-establish and maintain a weight pattern above the third centile, then Study 1 showed that children diagnosed as organic, non-organic and 'small' stood a roughly equal chance of improvement. This suggests that indicators of poverty and deprivation have little impact on whether a child gets better or continues to fail to thrive. We also found, as have other studies, that children who were premature or have been admitted to a special care baby unit are at risk of poor weight gain but, in terms of outcome, they were no more likely to fall into the category Non-Improver than into the category Improver.

However, we also found in Study 1 that a small number of children were admitted to hospital for investigation of low weight, and that when this admission was accompanied by weight gain whilst in hospital the child was highly likely to continue to fail to thrive on discharge. This suggested that feeding behaviour was a central issue for children who did not improve. From this we hypothesised that feeding problems would discriminate between those children whose episode below the third centile was one-off and brief and those whose episode was long-lasting or recurrent, placing them at risk of delayed or permanently impaired development. The limited data on feeding problems in Study 1 supported this hypothesis, so Study 2 was designed to focus on such problems.

In Study 2 we did not use health visitor recall to obtain our sample, but examined 6-8,000 child health clinic cards and about 2,000 health visitor notes to identify children below the third centile and to extract data on them. We found that for every two children recognised by health visitors as low weight gainers, one passed unrecognised despite the child's weights being entered onto the health records. We also found there were often long gaps between weights being taken, that they were sometimes recorded inaccurately or imprecisely, that centile charts were often incomplete and that there was no easy system for retrieving records of children who had been below the third centile.

We investigated feeding in Study 2 and found that the number of feeding problems did discriminate between those we categorised as Non-Improvers and Improvers, although this relationship only held for children recognised by health visitors as low weight gainers. In examining the distribution of feeding problems amongst those recognised as low weight gainers, we found a difference across the outcome categories. The number of problems recorded was not just a reflection of the child's low weight having been recognised but rather was directly related to the severity of problems experienced by parents.

Allowing for health visitor non-recognition of children in Study 1, and excluding children constantly below the third centile from birth and those with specific growth-limiting syndromes, we estimate that about 150 children under five in the district in which the two studies were conducted were failing to thrive in 1987. Thus over 1% of the under-fives population was below the third centile for weight, having previously established a growth pattern above this. This is less than the 3% one might expect by virtue of the way centile charts are constructed. However, we have confined ourselves to those children who dropped to this centile position, excluding those below the third centile from birth. We also know that, in addition to its relative value, a weight below the third centile on the charts used in child health clinics in Britain is low in absolute terms. Using the example of a girl aged one year, the 50th centile weight is 9.8 kg. whilst the 3rd centile weight is only 7.8 kg, 80% of the 50th centile weight. The difference between the 3rd and 50th centile is wide.

We began this paper by arguing that failure to thrive has been lost from the child welfare agenda. We believe that our research shows some of the consequences of this lack of attention. It might be argued that it is appropriate that failure to thrive should not receive as much attention as some other child care issues. Few children die as a result of the condition. In addition, the literature on failure to thrive is somewhat inconclusive when it comes to specifying the extent to which long term effects are influenced by such factors as the child's age at onset. However, set against this imprecision is the knowledge that sustained failure to thrive does have long term consequences, many of which may not be immediately apparent in childhood. It may indicate serious social or medical problems that require speedy intervention.

Health visitors weigh young children in the course of conducting child health clinics. This practice is likely to continue so long as parents and health visitors find it valuable, despite some doubts regarding the effectiveness of this surveillance (Butler 1989). The use of centile charts by health visitors is already widely encouraged and recommended (Hall 1989). This should ensure that children who are failing to thrive are identified. Yet from our studies we know that one third of children whose weights fall below the third centile are not recognised as such by health visitors. If every child had all their weights entered onto a centile chart, all children falling below the third centile could be speedily identified.

Even when children are identified as failing to thrive, the range of interventions available is limited. We have argued that low weight gain, leading to children spending a sustained period of time below the third centile, is often perpetuated by feeding difficulties, irrespective of what started the failure to thrive. The literature suggests that feeding problems are open to intervention, and there is scope for development of projects to provide effective treatment.

The term 'failure to thrive' is used very broadly. It is our impression from discussions with health and social services staff that the term has different meanings for different people. For many health visitors children were only cases of failure to thrive when they were suffering from neglect in addition to low weight gain. This might be one factor that contributes to health visitors not keeping accurate, up-to-date charts on all children, despite charts being available and their use being encouraged. In this respect, health visitor records do not differ greatly from those of social workers, whose records also frequently fail to meet with recommended practice guidelines (Kerslake and Cramp 1988). Health visitors operate as autonomous professionals, with a high degree of discretion regarding the manner in which they fulfil their duties. When under pressure from large caseloads, high staff turnover and low levels of administrative support, health visitors may be selective in their completion of charts. Under such conditions health visitors are likely to concentrate on children suffering from deprivation or neglect; that is, those fitting the traditional diagnosis of non-organic failure to thrive.

Finally, how do we move forward and build on our findings? There appear to be two important areas for further work. The first relates to our need for more research on the outcome for children who have failed to thrive. A starting point might be secondary analysis of data already held on some of the large scale longitudinal studies being conducted in Britain. Such analysis could extend our knowledge of the long term consequences of failure to thrive in early childhood. In addition, projects set up to target interventions for children failing to thrive should be closely monitored and evaluated.

The second, and perhaps most important, area for further research relates to our findings regarding the level of identification of children failing to thrive. Health visitors regularly weigh young children; they know the importance of identifying those who fall onto the third centile. Yet we found in our second study that for every two children identified as low weight gainers, and so monitored or referred to a specialist, one low weight gaining child was weighed and yet passed unrecognised. As our work has been based on one district health authority it is important that further work is done to replicate the studies. If our results hold across the country, thousands of children who are failing to thrive are not being detected, despite being weighed by health visitors. There would be value in nationwide research to examine the role of health visitors in relation to failure to thrive. This might include access to effective weighing equipment. However, what is most needed is an understanding of the factors that stop health visitors from fulfilling their duties for all children who are failing to thrive, and what can be done to improve rates of identification. We can then perhaps ensure that failure to thrive does not disappear from the child welfare agenda, and that these children receive the attention and treatment their condition merits.

References

BARKER, D. J. P. & OSMOND, C. (1987) 'Inequalities in Health in Britain: Specific Explanations in Three Lancashire Towns', British Medical Journal 294 pp749-752.

BECKFORD Report (1985) A Child in Trust: The Report of the Panel of Inquiry into the Circumstances Surrounding the Death of Jasmine Beckford (London Borough of Brent).

BITHONEY, W. G. & NEWBERGER, E. H. (1987) 'Child and Family Attributes of Failure-to-Thrive', Developmental and Behavioural Paediatrics 8(1) pp32-36.

BRIEND, A. & BARI, A. (1989) 'Critical Assessment of the Use of Growth Monitoring for Identifying High Risk Children in Primary Health Care Programmes', British Medical Journal 298 pp1607-1611.

BUTLER, J. (1989) Child Health Surveillance in Primary Care: A Critical Review (London: HMSO).

CARLILE Report (1987) A Child in Mind: Protection of Children in a Responsible Society. The Report of the Commission of Inquiry into the Circumstances Surrounding the Death of Kimberley Carlile (London Borough of Greenwich).

CENTRAL STATISTICAL OFFICE (1989) Annual Abstract of Statistics (London:HMSO)

CHATOOR, I., DICKSON, L., SCHAEFER, S. & EGAN, J. (1985) 'A Developmental Classification of Feeding Disorders Associated with Failure to Thrive: Diagnosis and Treatment', in Drotar, D. (ed) New Directions in Failure to Thrive: Implications for Research and Practice (Plenum Press), pp235-258.

DROTAR, D. (1985) 'Research and Practice in Failure to Thrive: the State of the Art', Zero to Three (Bulletin of the National Centre for Clinical Infant Programs) 5(3) pp1-4.

DROTAR, D., WOYCHIK, J., MANTZ-CLUMPNER, C., BRICKELL, C., NEGRAY, J., WALLACE, M. & MALONE, C. (1985) 'The Family Context of Failure to Thrive', in Drotar, D. (ed) New Directions in Failure to Thrive: Implications for Research and Practice (Plenum Press), pp295-310.

FARNAROFF & KLAUS (1972) 'Follow-up of Low Birth Weight Infants: Predictive Value of Maternal Visiting Patterns', Pediatrics 49 pp287-290.

FORFAR, J. & ARNEIL, G., (eds.) (1984) Textbook of Paediatrics Volume 1, pp475-479 (3rd Edition).

FRANK, D. A. et al (1985) 'Primary Prevention of Failure to Thrive: Social Policy Implications', Zero to Three (Bulletin of the National Centre for Clinical Infant Programs) 5(3) pp4-10.

GAGAN, R. J. et al (1984) 'The Families of Children who Fail to Thrive: Preliminary Investigations of Parental Deprivation among Organic and Non- organic Cases', Child Abuse and Neglect 8 pp93-103.

GOLDSON, E. (1986) 'Failure to Thrive: an Old Problem Revisited', in MacFarlane, J. A. (ed) Progress in Child Health 3 pp83-99.

HALL, D. M. B. (ed) (1989) Health for All Children: A Programme for Child Health Surveillance (Oxford Medical Publications).

HAYNES, C. et al (1983) 'Non-organic FTT: Decisions for Placement and Videotaped Evaluations', Child Abuse and Neglect 7 pp309-319.

HAYNES, C. F., CUTLER, C., GRAY, J. & KEMPE, R. S. (1984) 'Hospitalized Cases of Nonorganic Failure to Thrive: The Scope of the Problem and Short-Term Lay Health Visitor Intervention', Child Abuse & Neglect 8 pp229-242.

HUFTON, I. & OATES, R. (1977) 'Nonorganic Failure To Thrive: A Long Term Follow-up', Paediatrics 59(1) pp73-77.

ILLINGWORTH, R. S. (1983) The Development of the Infant and Young Child (8th Edition).

IWANIEC, D. (1987) 'Assessment and Treatment of Failure-to-Thrive Children and their Families', The Behavioural Social Work Review Summer 1987 8(2a) pp9-19.

IWANIEC, D., HERBERT, M. & MCNEISH, A.S. (1985) 'Social Work with Failure-to-Thrive Children and their Families - Part I: Psychosocial Factors', British Journal of Social Work 15 pp243-259.

IWANIEC, D., HERBERT, M. & MCNEISH, A.S. (1985b) 'Social Work with Failure-to-Thrive Children and their Families - Part II: Behavioural Social Work Intervention', British Journal of Social Work 15 pp375-389.

IWANIEC, D., HERBERT, M. & SLUCKIN, A. (1988) 'Helping Emotionally Abused Children Who Fail to Thrive', in Browne, K., Davies, C. & Stratton, P. (eds) Early Prediction and Prevention of Child Abuse (Wiley & Sons) pp 229-244.

JONES, D. N., PICKETT, J., OATES, M. R. & BARBOR, P. (1987) Understanding Child Abuse 2nd edition (London: Macmillan Education).

KARNISKI, W., VAN BUREN, L. & CUPOLI, J. M. (1986) 'A Treatment Program for Failure to Thrive: A Cost/Effectiveness Analysis', Child Abuse & Neglect 10 pp471-478.

KERSLAKE, A. & CRAMP, J. (1988) A New Child Care Model: The Evidence for Change (Bath Social Policy Paper No. 14, University of Bath).

KOTELCHUCK, M. (1980) 'Nonorganic Failure to Thrive: the Status of Interactional and Environmental Etiologic Theories', in Camp, B. (ed) Advances in Behavioural Pediatrics, Volume 1 (Greenwich: JAI Press).

LACHENMEYER, J. & DAVIDOVICZ, H. (1987) 'Failure to Thrive: A Critical Review', Advancement of Clinical Child Psychology 10 pp335-358.

LAKING, P. (1988) 'Appearances can be Deceptive', Community Care (Feb 25th) 700 pp26-27.

LOBSTEIN, T. (1988) 'Poor Children and Cheap Calories', Community Paediatric Group Newsletter August 1988 pp4-5 (British Paediatric Association).

MacCARTHY, D. (1974) 'Effects of Emotional Disturbance and Deprivation on Somatic Growth', in Davis, J. and Dobbing, J. (eds) Scientific Foundations of Paediatrics pp56-67.

MITCHELL, W. G. et al (1980) 'Failure-to-Thrive: A Study in a Primary Care Setting. Epidemiology and Follow-up', Pediatrics 65(5) pp971-977.

MOORE, J. (1982) 'Project Thrive: A Supportive Treatment Approach to the Parents of Children with Nonorganic Failure to Thrive', Child Development 61(6) pp389-398.

O'NEILL Report (1945) Report by Sir Walter Monckton on the circumstances which led to the boarding out of Dennis and Terence O'Neill at Bank Farm, Misterley and the steps taken to supervise their welfare (London: HMSO).

OATES, R. K. (1984) 'Similarities and Differences between Nonorganic Failure to Thrive and Deprivation Dwarfism', Child Abuse and Neglect 8 pp439-445.

PACEY, A. & PAYNE, P. (eds) (1985) Agricultural Development and Nutrition (Hutchinson).

POLLITT, E., EICHLER, A. & CHAN, C. (1975) 'Psychosocial Development and Behaviour of Mothers of Failure-to-Thrive Children', American Journal of Orthopsychiatry 45(4) pp525-537.

PRADER, A. (1978) 'Catch Up Growth', in Barltrop, D. (ed) Paediatrics and Growth (Fellowship of Postgraduate Medicine) pp133-146.

SKUSE, D. (1985) 'Non-organic Failure to Thrive: A Reappraisal', Archives of Disease in Childhood 60 pp173-178.

SKUSE, D. (1988) 'Failure to Thrive: Failure to Feed', Community Paediatric Group Newsletter August 1988 pp6-7 (British Paediatric Association).

SMITHELLS, R. W. (1982) 'In Praise of Outpatients: Partnership in Paediatrics', in Apley, J. and Ounsted, C. (eds) One Child.

TANNER, J.M. & WHITEHOUSE, R. H. (1959) 'Standards for Height and Weight of British Children from Birth to Maturity', Lancet 2 pp1086-1088.

TAYLOR, C. E. & TAYLOR, E. M. (1976) 'Multi-factorial Causation of Malnutrition', in McClaren D. (ed) Nutrition in the Community (Wiley & Sons).

WINICK, M. (1980) Nutrition in Health and Disease (Wiley & Sons).

Appendix I

STUDY 1: QUESTIONNAIRE A
HEALTH VISITOR INTERVIEWS

HEALTH VISITOR ....   AREA.........................
DATE.........

GENERAL INFORMATION ON CASELOAD:

1. Caseload: number of families with children
under 5 in 1987.   NUMBER...............

2. Caseload: number of children under 5 in 1987.
                                         NUMBER................

3. Number of children under 5 on Child Protection
Register in 1987.   NUMBER...............

4. Number of Priority Cases in 1987.   NUMBER...............

5. Number of children under 5 on H/Vs caseload in
1987 who were on or below the 3rd centile for
weight gain.   NUMBER...............

6. Number of children under 5 on H/Vs caseload in
1987 who were causing her concern because of
developmental delay.   NUMBER...............

7. Number of children under 5 on H/Vs caseload in
1987 who were causing her concern because of low
clinic attendance and/or poor use of health
facilities.   NUMBER...............

8. To what extent do children in Questions 5, 6
and 7 overlap.

RESOURCES FOR FTT CHILDREN:

1. What avenues exist in this area for referral ofSPECIFY...........
children thought to be failing to thrive, other ....
than those covered in B.   ....

2. Why were these avenues not used in the above   REASONS...........
cases.   ....

3. What other forms of treatment exist in this   SPECIFY...........
area for children thought to be failing to   ....
thrive, other than those covered in B.   ....

4. Why were these not used in the above cases.   REASONS...........
                                                   ....

5. What additional resources would the H/V find   SPECIFY...........
useful in her work with children who are   ....
 failing to thrive and their families.   ....

6. What access does the H/V have to scales.   DETAILS...........
                                                   ....

INFORMATION ON H/V AND HER WORKING ENVIRONMENT:

1. How many years has the H/V been qualified.   ....YEARS

2. Any additional training since her Health   NO / YES
Visitor qualification.   (specify).........
                                                   ....

3. How many years has she been working in her   ....YEARS
present post.

4. What geographical area does she cover.   TOWN/LOCALITY.......
                                                   ....
5. How would she descibe the area she covers.   TOWN/VILLAGES/ RURAL
                                                   OTHER(specify).......

6. What types of housing predominate   OWNER OCCUPIER/
in the area she covers.   COUNCIL/RENTED
                                                   PRIVATE/TIED /OTHER
                                                   (specify.........)/NK

7. How would the H/V rate the channels of
communication with her professional colleagues:
a) H/V and GPs   GOOD/ADEQUATE/POOR/NONE
b) H/V and CMO   GOOD/ADEQUATE/POOR/NONE
c) H/V and paediatrician/s   GOOD/ADEQUATE/POOR/NONE
d) H/V and Social Services   GOOD/ADEQUATE/POOR/NONE
e) H/V and her supervisor/manager   GOOD/ADEQUATE/POOR/NONE
f) H/V and other professionals;
 specify.........   GOOD/ADEQUATE/POOR/NONE

Appendix II

STUDY 1: QUESTIONNAIRE B
FOR SPECIFIC INFORMATION ON 'FTT' CHILDREN

For each child under 5 identified by health visitor as on/below 3rd
centile for weight in 1987:
CHILD'S NAME.................
CODE.................

Is/was the child:
On the Child Protection Register: NOT KNOWN / NO / YES........
A Priority Case: NOT KNOWN / NO / YES........
Developmentally delayed: NOT KNOWN / NO / YES........
Low clinic attender: NOT KNOWN / NO / YES........

1. Child's month and year of birth.   ..... / ....

2. Child's birth weight, head, length. WEIGHT.....................
                                        HEAD CIRCUMFERENCE.........
                                        LENGTH.....................

3. Child's sex.   MALE / FEMALE

4. Child's racial/ethnic origin.   SPECIFY....................

5. Age of child when FTT first suspected...........MONTHS

6. Household composition at that time. TWO PARENTS / SINGLE PARENT /
                                        STEPFAMILY / OTHER.........

7. This child's position in family,   1 / 2 / 3 / 4 / 5 / 6......
when FTT first suspected.
(Circle position & delete figures to show number of children in
household)

8. Any cot deaths in this family.   NOT KNOWN / NO / YES (date..)

9. Where child lived in 1987.   TOWN / VILLAGE / RURAL
                                          ADDRESS....................

10. Type of accommodation in 1987.   OWNER OCCUPIER / COUNCIL / RENTED
                                        PRIVATE / TIED / OTHER
                                        (specify........) / NOT KNOWN

11. Any major changes in child's family since FTT concern. (Eg death, divorce, move of house, birth of sibling, illness, unemployment)
....

12. Was a parent or stepparent with whom the child lived in 1987 in full time employment.   YES / NO / NOT KNOWN

13. If yes, nature of employment
of chief earner.   MANUAL / NON MANUAL / NOT KNOWN

14. Who first expressed concern re child's slow growth or poor weight gain.
PARENT/HEALTH VISITOR/GP/CMO/PAEDIATRICIAN/SOCIAL WORKER/OTHER...../NOT KNOWN

15. Was poor weight gain initially picked up at the child's developmental check.   YES / NO / NOT KNOWN

16. Did H/V refer the child to another professional because of FTT.
YES / NO

17. If H/V did refer the child on, where did she refer her/him.
GP / CMO / PAEDIATRICIAN / SOCIAL WORKER / OTHER
(specify...................)

18. What factors influenced the H/V's decision WHETHER to refer or not.
SPECIFY...

19. What factors influenced the H/V's decision re WHERE to refer.
SPECIFY...

20. What was the course of events after initial concern (include action by health visitor, GP, CMO, paediatrician etc), including approximate time scale.
DRAW TIME CHART
INCLUDE APPOINTMENTS OFFERED BUT NOT KEPT.

21. What was outcome of any referral, in terms of:
a) identification of cause of FTT.

ORGANIC / NON ORGANIC /'SMALL CHILD'/
OTHER (specify........) / NOT KNOWN

b) treatment.

HOSPITAL IN-PATIENT /
OUTPATIENT / HV MONITORS / OTHER
(specify.............) / NOT KNOWN

22. What is the current situation regarding this child's growth.
CONTINUOUS FTT
IMPROVED THEN RELAPSE
IMPROVED
OTHER (specify..............)
NOT KNOWN

23. Has the H/V completed centile charts for this child's:
a) weight (naked?),   NO / YES (date/s...........)
b) height,   NO / YES (date/s...........)
c) head circumference. NO / YES (date/s...........)

24. Has any other child in this family been investigated for FTT.
NOT KNOWN / NO / YES (details.......
.............................)

Appendix III

DISTRICT HEALTH AUTHORITY NOTES FOR HEALTH VISITORS

PRIORITY FAMILIES

Guidelines towards Identifying Factors

1. Poor bonding with either parent

2. Single parent family, either parent

3. Parent known to have previous history of:

    a) child abuse, actual or suspected;
    b) known criminal record;
    c) neglect, actual or suspected.

4. Very young parent(s)

5. Large number of pregnancies/siblings (if other factors present)

6. Marital problems

7. Financial problems

8. Unemployment

9 Poor housing

10. Emotional deprivation

11. Social

12. Medical